Dr M

DR MIKE SMITH cine, a practising GP, medical writer. He was the Chief Medical Officer of the Family Planning Association 1970–75 and their Honorary Medical Adviser 1975–90. For many years he has been a 'resident' expert guest on BBC2's Jimmy Young Programme and was LBC's regular broadcasting doctor from its inception and continues with its successor, London News Talk Radio. He has been seen and heard on most TV channels and radio stations throughout the British Isles over the last 25 years. In April 1991, he was voted the TV and Radio Doctors' 'Expert's Expert' in the *Observer* magazine's series.

His other books include *Birth Control*, *How to Save Your Child's Life*, *A New Dictionary of Symptoms*, *Dr Mike Smith's Handbook of Over-The-Counter Medicines*, *Dr Mike Smith's First Aid Handbook* and *Dr Mike Smith's Handbook of Prescription Medicine*.

Also in *Dr Mike Smith's Postbag* series:

Allergies

Arthritis

Back-Pain

Eating Disorders

HRT

Infertility

Migraine

Skin Problems

Stress

DR MIKE SMITH'S POSTBAG

ASTHMA

WITH SHARRON KERR

KYLE CATHIE LIMITED

Copyright © Dr Mike Smith 1995

All rights reserved. No reproduction, copy or transmission of this publication may be made without written permission. No paragraph of this publication may be reproduced, copied or transmitted save with written permission or in accordance with the Copyright Act 1956 (as amended). Any person who does any unauthorised act in relation to this publication may be liable to criminal prosecution and civil claims for damages.

Dr Mike Smith is hereby identified as the author of this work in accordance with Section 77 of the Copyright, Designs and Patents Act 1988.

First published 1995 by
Kyle Cathie Limited
20 Vauxhall Bridge Road
London SW1V 2SA

ISBN 1 85626 196 4

A CIP catalogue record for this title
is available from the British Library

Typeset in Palatino by
SX Composing Ltd, Rayleigh, Essex
Printed and bound by Cox & Wyman Ltd, Reading, Berks

CONTENTS

Introduction	1
What is Asthma?	3
The signs and symptoms of asthma	4
What causes asthma?	4
How is asthma diagnosed?	7
The treatment of asthma	7
How to cope with an attack	12
When does asthma become an emergency?	15
Asthma and Childhood	20
Common Asthma Triggers	30
The house dust mite	30
Pollution	32
Asthma and exercise	39
Asthma, stress and emotions	45
Asthma and smoking	48
Pollen	54
Asthma and infections	58
Asthma and other medicines	58
How to Deal with your Doctor	60
Prevention and Self-help Treatment	67
Going on Holiday	76
Asthma and Pregnancy	77

Alternative Treatments	81
Acupuncture	82
Homoeopathy	83
Herbal Medicine	84
Reflexology	85
Yoga	86
Alexander Technique	86
Osteopathy	86
Chiropractic	87
Common Questions	89
Asthma Research	99
Useful Addresses	100
Index	102

INTRODUCTION

Effortless breathing is something we take very much for granted. If any disorder affects the lungs or breathing tubes – the bronchial spasm of asthma, for example – breathing in and out can become a frightening effort. Millions of people in this country know just what that experience of breathing difficulty is like. In fact, in the UK it is thought that some three million people suffer from asthma and that it accounts for approximately 100,000 hospital admissions each year. Asthma does vary in severity and most sufferers will have fairly mild symptoms for most of the time. But even so attacks can hit them right out of the blue, leaving them gasping and fighting for air.

Treatment has improved over recent years and most patients can expect to lead normal and active lives by managing their asthma responsibly and with the full help of their doctor or, increasingly, their asthma clinic nurse.

I am often asked about asthma by my readers and listeners. The questions are mainly from the mothers of children who have recently been diagnosed. They are often surprised that what seemed to them to be a 'weak chest' should have been diagnosed as asthma and their main concern is whether it is likely to be a life-long illness. Once a label has been attached to symptoms it can be a comfort to some sufferers but a definite worry to others. Generally I can reply that many children who have asthma in their childhood will fortunately be relieved of their symptoms as they grow

– as I explain later. And I also explain that asthma is a collection of symptoms and not a specific illness. It does not have one single cause or trigger. In some sufferers with one main trigger, often a food, it may be possible to avoid that trigger and thus avoid the symptoms of asthma.

The other main concern that I am asked about is the likely effect of taking steroids – whether from an inhaler or, in the case of more serious asthma sufferers, larger doses by mouth. The amount taken in inhalers is very small but highly effective. An occasional infection – with thrush, for example – in the mouth or throat is the most common 'side-effect'. If the steroids have to be taken in tablet form, the minimum dose that controls the symptoms will soon be achieved, even in the more severe of attacks. At these levels the side-effects of weight gain and water retention can be kept to a minimum. And it must be remembered that without such steroids – indeed only in recent decades, before they were available – an asthma attack was a much greater danger than it is now, and all too often had tragic results.

This book is not intended as a D-I-Y diagnosis tool or in any way to replace medical consultation or advice from your GP or asthma clinic nurse. My aim is to help you understand your asthma in order that you can take an active, informed part in its day-to-day management. In the following chapters I aim to explain simply and clearly what asthma is, how it can be treated, what the most common triggers are, how to cope with an attack, what alternative therapies might offer and I talk to sufferers who give a clear picture of what living with asthma is really like.

WHAT IS ASTHMA?

So what exactly is asthma? Put simply it is an inflammatory condition that causes a swelling of the lining membrane of the breathing tubes, thus constricting them. At the same time, the very small muscles in these tubes contract, narrowing them even further. Too much mucus is produced, which makes the tubes effectively even narrower still.

Normally we breathe air – containing life-giving oxygen – in through our nose and mouth and it reaches our lungs via the trachea (windpipe) which branches into two bronchi, one bronchus serving each lung. The bronchi themselves divide many times into smaller and smaller tubes, called bronchioles, which end in tiny airsacs, which in turn transfer oxygen into the main bloodstream to be carried throughout the body. In exchange, the unwanted carbon-dioxide gas from the blood is breathed out.

These bronchial tubes are not rigid but widen and narrow. They are narrower when we breathe out than they are when we breathe in. In asthma, when the airways narrow, it is more difficult for the air to get in and out. That's why asthma symptoms – that feeling of shortness of breath, the wheezing, coughing and feelings of tightness in the chest – are experienced. And that's why you can hear wheezing, mainly as you breathe out, because air is being forced out through very narrow tubes. Sticky phlegm (sputum) is also produced which is coughed up or which makes you feel as though your chest is congested.

THE SIGNS AND SYMPTOMS OF ASTHMA

Symptoms may be one or any of the following: chest 'tightness', a shortness of breath, or a wheeze or a cough. You don't have to experience all the symptoms all together to suffer from asthma.

Asthma symptoms are worse at some times than at others because the swelling of the lining tissues waxes and wanes throughout the day. Consequently, the obstruction of airflow is variable – and it is this variation which is the main characteristic of asthma.

The symptoms of a severe attack can also include: a severe shortness of breath – often the patient will seem to be fighting to breathe – paleness in the face, an inability to speak, as well as exhaustion.

When people suffer from asthma, they can experience a huge difference in symptoms from individual to individual. One person may only be aware of a slight wheeze, whereas others may find their asthma is so severe it imposes restraints on their life. Some may need repeated admission to hospital. But, in fact, most people who have asthma will have mild symptoms for a large part of the time, interspersed infrequently with more serious asthma attacks.

WHAT CAUSES ASTHMA?

Anyone who doesn't know much about asthma may find it surprising that this problem can be allergy-related. In fact, one of the most common causes of asthma attacks is an allergy, usually to house-dust mites, pollen, feathers or animals.

But how can an allergic reaction end up in an asthma attack? An allergy is the result of the body's defence mechanism going into top gear. An allergen is any substance in the environment which when taken into the body may cause it to become hypersensitive. The body can over-react when harmless substances, such as pollen in the air or pet hairs, are 'viewed' by the body's defence system (antibodies) as foreign. The antibodies in the sufferer's blood – produced to protect us from germs – may then react to the allergen, releasing powerful chemicals which cause the symptoms of the allergy, a spasm of the bronchial muscles (asthma), or excessive secretions in the nose or eyes, or a skin rash. (Tests show that those prone to an allergy tend to have a much higher concentration of one particular type of antibody in their blood known as immunoglobulin E – IgE for short.)

The antibodies attack our mast cells (large cells found in the skin, nose, lungs and intestines), releasing the chemical histamine and at least seven other substances which cause the tiny blood vessels (capillaries) to dilate and their walls to leak. Of course, when an infection is the cause this is good for the body as the dilated blood vessels bring in more blood cells and antibodies to deal with the invaders and the secretion dilutes the infectious agent to help wash it out of the nose, for example.

An allergic reaction can take many guises. Sufferers can experience difficulties in breathing as those encountered in an asthma attack; bouts of sneezing, itchy eyes, eczema and even migraine are some other examples.

But allergy is not the only thing that can set off an asthma attack. Chest infections can also trigger asthma. In adults, attacks are not necessarily caused by an allergy, but by one of many other triggers such as an over-reaction of the lung-lining tissues to cold temperatures, for example, or to exercise. In someone who suffers from asthma, worry and anxiety, perhaps caused by pressure at work or at home, or exposure to air pollution, can make the condition worse. Asthma is often more than a physical condition; it can be a social one as well, with attacks induced by emotion – even simple things such as laughter or excitement can bring on the symptoms.

Recently, scientists have been looking at the link between genetic factors and asthma. There are likely to be some genetic associations, at least for certain types of sufferers. When asthma 'runs in the family' it is usually associated with a higher level than usual of a certain type of body defence – a group of antibodies. In sufferers this is present in a higher concentration than in the rest of the population. I believe that this will be linked to an inherited gene as the genetic puzzles that exist at present are unravelled by the doctors and research scientists. And some time after that, as with so many other conditions which ail us, we may well be able to do something beneficial to the offending genes themselves.

For many asthmatics the cause remains a mystery – it is just something they have to live with. One of the problems with asthma is that symptoms can come on very suddenly and can cause great distress. Fortunately, though, most people can learn to control their asthma by taking the correct medication and by learning not to panic when they feel an attack coming on.

HOW IS ASTHMA DIAGNOSED?

Doctors will usually be able to tell by listening to an account of your symptoms whether asthma is likely. Very often asthma medicines will be prescribed to see whether they have an impact on symptoms, particularly when a young child is involved.

A doctor may decide to monitor older children's and adults' breathing by using peak flow meter readings (see also page 74) to help ascertain whether the asthma improves with medication. A peak flow meter is a simple gauge which, when you blow as hard as you can, helps you measure the peak expiratory flow, which is a very good indicator of how well your lungs are functioning. Remember, one of the characteristics of asthma is that the obstruction to the bronchial tubes caused by the inflammation of their lining and the contraction of their wall muscles is reversible – it comes and goes. Consequently the peak flow readings which measure these restrictions will differ throughout the day. In someone who doesn't have asthma the readings will usually be constant. As a result, the history of the chest symptoms, the doctor's examination of the sufferer's chest, together with the peak flow readings will usually allow a doctor to be confident about making a diagnosis of asthma.

THE TREATMENT OF ASTHMA

Asthma can be treated readily and effectively. If diagnosed, your doctor will probably prescribe an inhaler which projects the medication into the area where it is most needed – the breathing passages.

Medicines are given to help prevent the symptoms occurring or to give relief, or both. Remember that in all cases of asthma, whatever the cause, drugs can be used to great effect. The medicines used to treat asthma include bronchodilators (airway openers) – called relievers – and inhaled steroids to help dampen down the inflammation and irritability of the airways – called preventers.

The major bronchodilators are salbutamol (Ventolin, for example) and terbutaline (Bricanyl), best taken by inhaler (or in the form of an aerosol mist by a nebuliser), because this means that small amounts of medicine reach the airways quickly to relax muscle spasm.

You may also be prescribed bronchodilators in tablet or syrup form. Most common side-effects of salbutamol and terbutaline include mild muscle tremor (usually the hands), anxiety and restlessness, cramp and palpitations.

Theophylline is another kind of bronchodilator prescribed in capsule, tablet or syrup form (Lasma, for example) which relaxes bronchial muscles. The most common side-effects of theophylline include nausea or vomiting.

It is worthwhile pointing out that patients should be aware that the increasing need to use a 'relieving' inhaler to control a sufferer's symptoms is a reason for notifying the doctor, without undue delay, that the symptoms are getting worse. If they are ignored, a potentially dangerous deterioration of the asthma could occur and lead to a serious attack with all that this means – a hospital admission and a severely distressed sufferer and their family.

The emphasis these days in asthma management is on prevention. This attitude allows treatment to be increased and stepped up or cut down according to the severity of the asthma at the time.

The British Thoracic Society guidelines wisely recommend that asthma is managed in a stepwise manner. The guidelines emphasise 'stepped care' in managing patients with chronic persistent asthma. This important concept defines levels of treatment that should be increased to reflect the severity of the disease. The treatment 'steps' should be logical, orderly and consistent. The message is to 'go strong', and then decrease medication when control is achieved. The following management steps are recommended:

Step 1 The use of intermittent inhaled bronchodilators (i.e. reliever inhalers).
Step 2 The use of regular prophylactic anti-inflammatories (inhaled steroids are first choice).
Step 3 The use of high-dose inhaled corticosteroids.
Step 4 The use of additional bronchodilators (ipratropium, aminophylline, oral bronchodilators and nebulised therapy).
Step 5 The use of corticosteroids.

Inhaled steroids (Becloforte and Becotide, for example) are effective as they help dampen down the irritability of the airways. In standard doses there are relatively few side-effects because of the small size of the doses involved and because, when inhaled, the medicine goes straight away to the airways. This lowers the risk of the medicine affecting any other part of the body. Sometimes patients develop a mild throat infection, and occasionally others find that their voice becomes husky. It might help to rinse your mouth thoroughly with water after using such a medicine.

Steroids are near-relatives of many of the natural hormones produced in our body. For instance, our adrenal glands secrete them when we're injured or under stress and these hormones are natural, cortisone-type healing and calming agents. Other steroids are secreted internally to control the body's sexual functions.

The inhaled steroids used to treat asthma are called corticosteroids. Those taken – unofficially – by some sportspeople are called anabolic steroids. These can cause a temporary increase in the mass and tone of the muscles of the body, as well as the speed with which the muscles work.

Sodium cromoglycate (Intal, for example) is also used to prevent symptoms of asthma, and may halt the release of certain chemicals which cause spasm. It can also cause throat irritation, coughing and brief bronchospasm. Steroid tablets (Prednisolone, for example) may be needed for severe asthma. Oral steroids can be life-saving and tend to be used in the minimum dose which produces the desired effect. Fortunately, many sufferers will have their symptoms controlled sufficiently so that their dose of steroids can be reduced to a low maintenance level that won't increase their weight.

People become quite concerned about the thought of taking steroids and often raise the issue with me. They're worried about moving on to steroids and never being able to come off them again because of the many stories that they have heard about their side-effects. Such side-effects are fortunately uncommon in the doses needed to control most cases of asthma.

Nevertheless, some are very reluctant indeed to

use them. Yet the benefits of preventative therapy are immense. Taken regularly as directed by the doctor they keep the symptoms at bay and prevent the onset of a potentially life-threatening attack. Many sufferers understandably don't feel that it's right to take medicines when they feel perfectly well in themselves and, in spite of the doctor's instructions, will just leave them off. Once they find (though regrettably to their cost because a frightening attack hits them) that they cannot do without them, they will rarely stop them again until they are advised to do so – and then usually gradually – if it is considered that the risks have reduced: in a growing child, for example.

The small whole body doses received with inhaled steroids are quickly destroyed by the liver, unlike the larger doses received with oral steroids, and are far less likely to cause side-effects than many other drugs (see page 58).

Prevention makes you more in control of your asthma and its triggers, rather than the medicine being in control of you.

There are many different asthma medicines but in general when you are mildly or moderately affected by asthma you are likely to be prescribed an inhaled 'reliever' medicine called a beta-agonist, to be taken as needed, and an inhaled 'preventer' steroid morning and evening.

Inhalers have different devices to enable the most efficient administration of your particular medicine. They may be breath-activated, give metered doses, work with a Diskhaler, a Nebuhaler, a Rotahaler, a Spinhaler, a Turbohaler, or a Volumatic which is a large spacer device. Smaller spacers, together with masks, are available for young children.

Asthma medicines can be taken by means of a nebuliser, although this is only advisable if your doctor recommends it and you may find that you have to buy the equipment yourself as GPs aren't allowed to prescribe it on the NHS. A nebuliser is made up of a compressor, a nebuliser and a face-mask or mouthpiece which enables the drug to be taken by means of a fine mist which is inhaled directly into the lungs. The concentration of the drug in the blood stream, required for effective relief of the symptoms, can be achieved as quickly through nebulisers as by an intravenous injection. The lungs contain a very large area of breathing membrane which allows extremely quick absorption of the inhaled medicine, so nebulisers tend to be used to treat asthma emergencies by GPs, in ambulances and when a person is admitted to hospital, to enable large doses of medicines to be given quickly and efficiently.

Your asthma clinic nurse or practice nurse will be able to help you work out which type of device is most suited to you and she can offer advice on inhaler techniques. The needs will differ from individual to individual, both because of the differing seriousness of the asthma as well as their ability to cope with the techniques required by the inhaler. It can be very difficult to squeeze and thus activate the inhaler at just the right moment to coincide with the insuck of breath so that the ingredient reaches the lungs as it is meant to.

HOW TO COPE WITH AN ATTACK

One asthma sufferer told me that advice on coping with an asthma attack was easy to administer, but not so easy to carry out.

WHAT IS ASTHMA?

It's very easy for someone who has never experienced an asthma attack to tell you to keep calm. I know some asthma sufferers who describe an attack as if there was a heavy weight on their chest or as if they are being strangled. But after an asthma attack, you realise that it must be a sensation that's the nearest thing to being buried alive. You're conscious of the fact that you are alive but at the same time you feel as if you are being suffocated and you can't do anything about it.

The only thing you can do is sit up straight and not move. By sitting still you're not exerting yourself or putting any pressure on yourself. Moving makes things even worse and makes it even more difficult to breathe. You do reach the stage sometimes when you can hardly breathe at all and then it's difficult to keep calm and try not to panic. Sometimes I know that I am trying to overbreathe, you know, taking lots of short, shallow breaths, the way someone having a panic attack does. I know too that panicking and breathing like this just makes the whole process even more frightening. The calmer you are the easier it is to keep the attack from escalating out of control so I do try as hard as I can to take slow deep breaths which does help me to relax.

Other asthma sufferers have told me that an attack can be so frightening and such 'hard work' that they get to the point where they don't care if they never take another breath of air again – a state of mind that could be very dangerous.

The basic aim of dealing with an asthma attack is obviously to help the sufferer start to breathe more easily again.

In a severe attack you will need to seek medical assistance by calling an ambulance immediately. While you are waiting for the ambulance to arrive, try to get the sufferer to take his or her medication, which should help any wheezing. They will have been told how to take it and how often. If, in the person's respiratory distress, he or she can barely speak – not at all uncommon in a severe attack – accept any refusal to follow your suggestions, as it may only make the sufferer more agitated if he or she does not have the breath to explain their reasons. Many sufferers have told me that often it is harder to deal with people fussing around them when they are having an attack than it is for them to concentrate on dealing with the attack. Most asthma sufferers will know exactly what they should do to keep calm and take their medication.

However, another action you can take is to help the sufferer into a comfortable position, for example, sitting up in a chair with hands on the knees, perhaps leaning slightly forward. A sufferer may take this position instinctively, as by so doing he or she is unconsciously anchoring the top ribs and so allowing the secondary muscles of respiration around the neck to be used to their best effect.

A severe asthma attack can be extremely frightening so you will need to appear calm (even if you are frightened too) until help arrives.

When an attack is less serious the sufferer still needs to take his or her medicine as soon as possible. If the attack does not respond to the usual treatment you must seek your doctor's advice. Each sufferer will usually know their own condition and how quickly their inhaler should bring them relief and when they need to take further action.

WHEN DOES ASTHMA BECOME AN EMERGENCY?

It is vitally important that the patient, relative or carer can recognise the severity of an attack. Always consult your doctor if you suspect the attack is severe as any delay could have serious consequences.

Asthma tragedies will best be reduced by recognising severe attacks and treating them aggressively. A potentially severe attack or increase in severity may be recognised by:

- The onset of a wheeze or difficulty with breathing so that the sufferer finds it difficult or impossible to speak or even move from where they are sitting.
- If the breathing rate increases to more than twenty-five breaths per minute.
- The pulse is constantly raised above 110 beats per minute.
- The peak flow meter reading is less than forty per cent of what it is, under normal circumstances, for that individual.

Awareness of the likely onset of an asthma attack from the criteria outlined above may prevent the development of a more serious attack. The most serious stage is recognised by the doctor by, for example, observing that:

- The top (systolic) blood pressure reading has now fallen by more than 10 mm as the sufferer sucks a breath in.

- The breath sounds that can usually be heard through a stethoscope on the sufferer's chest are much reduced or even almost absent.
- The heart has now slowed dangerously.
- The patient is going blue and is quite exhausted, confused or unconscious.

When emergency medical procedures are able to successfully treat such a severe attack it is absolutely essential that the patient is urgently reviewed, probably by a specialist, to make sure that the recommended medicines are taken regularly, or, if they are already being taken as prescribed, they are reassessed to prevent such a life-threatening attack from occurring again.

When Does Asthma Need Further Medication?

There are several signs which could mean your medication dosage needs to be changed or that you need further medication. Consult your doctor if you feel you are experiencing any of the following:

- If you find that you wake up at night feeling out of breath.
- If you notice you are more short of breath than usual when you get up in the morning.
- If you need your symptom-relieving medicines more and more and when you do take them they are not as effective as usual.
- If you use a peak flow meter and the differences between morning and evening readings are becoming more and more noticeable.
- If you are generally concerned that your asthma is deteriorating or, as one sufferer told me, 'If you feel things aren't as they should be or you can't do the things you are normally able to.'
- If a child sufferer often wakes at night coughing.

Why is Asthma Becoming More Common?

At the extreme end of the scale in Britain, about 2000 people a year die, and some others will tragically end up brain-damaged, as a result of a serious asthma attack. It is thought that forty per cent of the people who die from asthma are under retirement age. About half are over sixty-five. It is important, particularly for anxious parents, to remember that it is very rare for a child under the age of five to die as a result of an asthma attack.

More than one in ten of us suffer from some kind of asthma and it does seem to be on the increase. Some doctors believe, however, that more than a quarter of asthmatics continue to go undiagnosed.

The main reason why asthma is not suspected in such cases is because they don't have symptoms which worry them enough to go to the doctor, or they just put them down to a cold that's 'gone to the chest' or to a weak chest. The combination of a chest infection and other symptoms may mean that a sufferer, their parents, or even the doctor, may automatically consider it to be a follow-on from that chest infection. Sometimes it may be; but the possibility that it is asthma should always be considered and investigated.

Even so, asthma probably affects around three million people in the UK, a figure which includes more than a quarter of a million schoolchildren. One letter I received expressed surprise that when the writer's nine-year-old asthma-suffering son went on a school trip for the weekend, five other children in the group had to take their inhalers. Asthma affects about one child in ten, although some experts believe it could be even more than that and that it could affect around one in seven children. One of the worrying statistics I have read recently is that asthma is the only treatable condition in the Western world which is on the increase. There is no doubt either about its increase in the last thirty years, particularly among children.

No one really knows why, though some argue that specialists are simply spotting it more often. Often experts believe that the increase in air pollution – mainly from cars – could be a cause. Others point the finger at the rise in the numbers of house dust mites in our homes, thanks to better insulation, central heating and fitted carpets. I believe that it is likely to be a combination of factors.

According to the British Allergy Foundation, allergic asthma is five times more common in Australia than in Britain and twenty times more common in Britain than in China or Hong Kong. I can only guess as to why this should be so, but it is likely to be due to the differences in temperature between the countries – higher temperatures will increase the dispersal of pollen, while humidity will reduce it. In these countries the types of plants will differ too – for example, there may be fewer plants that rely on airborne pollen transport. Altitude may also have an effect: the higher land is dryer and so more conducive to pollen, the lower (especially Hong Kong at sea level) more humid and so less favourable to pollen dispersal. Pollution can also increase the incidence of asthma attacks. The body types of the people – Oriental Chinese compared with Caucasian Australians and British – are also likely to provoke different asthmatic responses.

People who know that their asthma is linked to allergy ask me whether or not we are developing more allergies. Some figures do suggest that over the last ten years more people are consulting their GP about these problems, in particular asthma and hayfever. There is the view that because, as a nation, we are becoming healthier, we are also becoming prone to allergic reactions from substances that might not have affected us before. It is suggested that as infectious diseases are brought under control in the developed world, our immune system starts to over-react to substances such as pollen, coming to identify them as harmful invaders, and treating them as if they were germs.

Does Asthma Run in Families?

Asthma can run in families but that does not mean to say that if you have asthma any child of yours will automatically develop it. For instance, if your family has a history of chest problems, eczema, hayfever or other specific allergies then there is more chance that someone in the family could develop asthma, although the extent to which they suffer from asthma is not passed on. This is known as a genetic predisposition.

ASTHMA AND CHILDHOOD

As with adult asthma, childhood asthma can vary dramatically in severity. A child may just experience bouts of mild wheezing when he or she has a cold, or have so many attacks of asthma that his or her development may be impaired.

The condition is often contracted quite young with symptoms mainly appearing by the age of five. Some surveys have shown that as many as eight out of ten children with asthma showed symptoms in the first two years of life.

It was always thought that most children would outgrow their asthma with the onset of puberty. Growing up probably helps because as the sufferer gets older, the main airways grow, which makes the air flow easier. But some doctors believe that it is not a question of outgrowing asthma but that children go into a stage of remission, which means that their asthma could be triggered again later on in life. One 1987 study highlighted the fact that of those children who suffered wheezing frequently when they were fourteen, marginally over two-thirds of them still had repeated bouts of asthma at the age of twenty-eight. Of those whose asthma had 'gone' by fourteen, nearly a third had recurrent symptoms when they were twenty-eight.

Yet, unfortunately, asthma is one of the most common chronic diseases of childhood in the Western world, making children prone to recurrent attacks of wheezing and breathlessness. In between attacks most children are as well as those who do not suffer from asthma.

ASTHMA AND CHILDHOOD 21

Between one in ten and one in seven children suffer from asthma and in children it affects twice as many boys as girls.

What are you most likely to notice in a child who shows symptoms of asthma for the first time? You should be suspicious if the child has more than the occasional cough, a wheeze at any time, or complains of breathlessness or whose breathing rate seems unduly rapid for the activity they are doing. Of course all these symptoms may be just that and due to an infection rather than diagnosable asthma – but it is wise to let your doctor be the judge of that, so do consult him.

The same trigger factors – allergy, a virus infection such as a cold or sore throat, emotions – apply to children as well as adults. Young children may come into contact with more virus infections at nursery and primary school and therefore are more likely to have their asthma triggered by these infections than adults. Once your child becomes older, possibly at around the age of six, he or she will be less prone, as any child, to virus infections as he or she will have come into contact with a wide range by now and so will have developed some immunity. As they develop their own antibodies to these early-met infections they will no longer catch them and their asthma from these triggers will be kept at bay as well.

Emotions can trigger off asthma attacks as much in children as in adults. Excitement, laughter, temper, frustration or family problems such as divorce can affect a child's emotions. One sufferer told me that her asthma was made worse by bottling up feelings when she was being bullied at school.

As for pets, it really does depend upon an individual child's response. If one of the strong triggers for the child's asthma is emotional upset, then the soothing pleasure that a pet can bring may actually improve the child's symptoms. However, if having an animal, particularly a cat, anywhere in the house triggers the asthma then it is likely that a goldfish or other non-triggering pet will have to be the alternative.

Dealing with a child's asthma attack is the same as dealing with an adult attack (see page 14), although as a parent you will probably need to stay even more calm so as not to panic your child.

The management of childhood asthma should promote the sufferer's participation in routine children's activities. Holding a child back will just isolate him or her and add to feelings that they are somehow different. This was often the usual approach to a child with asthma previously. As a result they missed much or most of their normal childhood so their lives and their potential were diminished. A child shouldn't be treated as an invalid. He or she shouldn't be omitted from school activities such as swimming, which is a good exercise – and particularly so for children – as it has been found to be less likely than other forms of exercise to provoke an asthma attack. The probable reasons for an attack while swimming is that the humidity close to the surface of the water entraps pollen and other dust allergens.

It is a good idea to let your child's school know about asthma problems so they are aware of any medication which needs to be taken.

The health professionals, together with the parents, have been making teachers aware of the essential – even vital – need for a child's access to their 'puffers'. As a result many if not most schools will now fully co-operate with medicine requirements. The few others who refuse to do so

ASTHMA AND CHILDHOOD 23

are putting the children in their care at considerable risk.

Try not to panic is one piece of advice Jackie, a thirty-nine-year-old accountant, would pass on to parents of children with asthma, even though at times it may be easier said than done. Her son Joseph had his first asthma attack when he was ten months old. She had no first-hand experience of asthma and didn't honestly realise the potential seriousness of the attack.

> I was at home on my own and he was obviously fighting for breath. Although I had a cousin who'd had asthma quite badly, I hadn't had first-hand experience of someone having an attack or what to do. I thought there must be something wrong but that it couldn't be as bad as I thought it was. You know how you always panic when a baby is not well. I kept thinking I'd wait for my husband to come home. In the end I phoned my mum up and she listened to the baby down the phone and told me to call the doctor out. It was a Sunday morning and obviously you don't want to call a doctor without good reason. He immediately said that he thought my son needed to go to hospital. My imagination ran wild, I didn't realise it was as serious as that.

That hospital admission was to be the first of many.

> I was very anxious that it would happen again and indeed he was in hospital about ten times in eighteen months. Looking back

on it, it was very hard for us as a family. But Joseph is much, much better now. At the time I didn't think about it very much but it was a difficult time because I have a daughter who's three years older and every time we had to rush off to the hospital I had to make arrangements for someone to look after her.

We have no idea what triggers his asthma. I got to the point where I was avoiding absolutely everything. I was sitting in the car avoiding having the windows open because of pollen. They say don't Hoover with them around – but what do you do with a toddler while you are Hoovering? I would put him in one room, Hoover the house quickly and then take him out in the car somewhere! It was very tricky.

I read about asthma. I picked up everything I could find on it. I got involved with the National Asthma Campaign and went to a few talks on asthma.

The advice I would give other parents is not to panic. You tend to panic and it is important not to over-react. You can make your lives absolutely miserable trying to find whatever it is that triggers the asthma and you can never get rid of everything that might be triggering it. And half the things you think of probably aren't triggering it in the first place.

Many parents have told me they blame themselves for their child's asthma. Virtually all good parents feel guilty about their children's suffering and think that at least they should be able to relieve it

ASTHMA AND CHILDHOOD 25

even if they don't really believe that they've caused it. My advice is that if you've done all you can to discover any triggers that can be avoided, do try not to blame yourself.

Jackie agrees that feeling guilty about your child having asthma is very unproductive.

> I did feel guilty. While I was pregnant I went on a photographic course and I was handling chemicals. I was convinced for a long time that it had to have something to do with that – although logic probably tells you it was nothing to do with it. You home in on these things when your child has asthma. I don't think you can let yourself feel guilty even if you think you brought it on your child genetically.

No matter how well you cope as a family with a child who has asthma, it still has some impact on family life.

> I suppose asthma has had an impact on our life because we have a boy and a girl and we may have had other children. But I had such a hard time with Joseph it did stop us having other children. I was pregnant again but had a miscarriage and after that we thought – no more. I used to be nebulising him four times a day for forty-five minutes at a time. Dealing with asthma in a young child takes up so much of your life and it also takes time away from the other children.

Joseph has not been admitted to hospital as a result of an asthma attack for two and a half years now although during that time he has been on quite high-dose steroids and, like many parents, Jackie was initially concerned about her son taking them.

> I was worried about him taking steroids. But then he has never shown any side-effects, any limiting of his growth and that sort of thing. He's over average height for his age, for instance. I'd rather have him take steroids than have an asthma attack – I've seen him blue in the face and almost being put on a ventilator. I don't worry about steroids and he is being weaned off them now. Prevention is better than having to deal with an attack.

Jackie also feels it's important that a parent of a child with asthma should keep his or her school closely informed about the extent of the asthma and what to do in an attack.

> When he goes to nursery, for instance, I make sure the teacher knows he should have his coat done up properly and shouldn't run around too much outside on cold, damp days, not to stop him playing or going outside, but just to be aware that he might react badly. Unless you spell out how the condition affects your child in particular, some teachers tend to slope off from it a bit. They are either frightened of it or they think it is not something as serious as it is. So I make sure I give staff as much information

as I can and tell them what to do in an emergency, or before they can get hold of me or a doctor.

Asthma sufferer Lisa, a twenty-one-year-old environmental management student, believes when a child has the condition, he or she should be kept well informed and any questions should be answered honestly.

> I don't think children should be treated as idiots. I'm not saying I was treated that way but I was only told what was thought I needed to know. Take this medicine and it will make you better, etc. If someone had sat me down and been honest with me and told me I'd have to take steroids preventatively but that I would not put on weight, or get blood clots, or have other side effects I would have taken them properly but I didn't until it was too late.
>
> I had a really bad attack when I was about seventeen. It was really, really frightening. If you can imagine how you feel when you're claustrophobic – you feel really enclosed and it's as if someone is putting their hand around your windpipe, making it get narrower and narrower and your breathing becomes shorter and shorter. When it's over you just feel such a sense of relief. But I feel if I had been told to take my medicines all the time because they were preventative it would have never happened.
>
> You can use asthma medicines to prevent the condition restricting you. If you let it rule

your life you're just in a negative cycle. Saying you can't exercise for example is a cop-out. There are Olympic swimmers who have asthma. I used to cycle a lot, I swim and I do step aerobics. I'm sure my asthma and my health are better for it – I enjoy it and it makes me stronger and fitter.

If you have asthma you should find out as much as you can about it and go to your asthma clinic and listen to what they have to say. Understanding asthma and its treatment is important in helping you cope.

When I was younger my asthma was really badly managed. If I don't use my preventer inhalers I have a bad attack. Pollen affects me badly. Last year when we had really high pollen levels I still had a bad attack but it's difficult to escape pollen.

My other triggers are cats, animal fur and pollution. I definitely think there's a link between asthma and pollution. Pollution is everywhere. Wherever you get people and cars, you are going to get pollution. I notice it most when I am sitting in a car in traffic. There might be a filthy lorry in front of me belching out smoke and I immediately begin to cough and my chest feels tight. It's not so bad when I'm walking down a busy street because I can get away from it. I also do feel better when I'm by the sea in Cornwall or Brighton. I don't know whether it's because there's less pollen by the sea.

While Lisa is now aware of some of her asthma trigger factors, she is equally aware of how she can live life within her own limitations by using her asthma medication effectively. But to do that she believes young people and children should understand what asthma is and how it, and the methods of controlling it, can affect their lives.

COMMON ASTHMA TRIGGERS

THE HOUSE DUST MITE

The house dust mite is a microscopic eight-legged 'beast' which lives – and thrives – on the dead skin cells that we shed constantly, particularly in bed. It is thought that we each shed approximately four pounds of these dead skin cells each year, so you can see the house dust mite's diet is in plentiful supply.

Each of these millions of mites produces twenty to forty faecal pellets a day – not a pretty thought! Fortunately, most of us co-exist quite happily with the mites, but the pellets are the trigger that provokes the allergic response and symptoms of perennial rhinitis in the susceptible. The faeces remain allergenic even after the mite that produced them has died, at the end of its three-to-four-month lifespan.

The trouble is caused by a digestive enzyme in these faeces, compounded by the fact that the faecal particles break down into very small pieces which are roughly the size of a grain of pollen. And just like pollen they are easily borne into the air, which is how they are inhaled or come into contact with skin. When inhaled the body's reaction, in those who are susceptible, is to treat the enzyme as an allergen and provoke an allergic reaction.

These mites are now thought to play a major role in allergies such as asthma, allergic rhinitis and eczema. One study carried out in the late 1980s showed that asthmatic patients demonstrated up to a forty per cent reduction in both asthma attacks and symptoms when they were moved to an environment which was mite-free. A later study carried out in Denmark showed that if a person had high levels of house dust mites in their homes they were five times more likely to suffer from eczema than those who lived in environments low in the mites.

The presence of dust mites in a home is not a reflection on the levels of cleanliness. House dust mites continue to thrive because modern conditions provide them with perfect breeding grounds. They love the warmth of our centrally heated homes and the humidity too, all contained within a modern house by properly fitted windows and doors, double glazing and house insulation. All those heat conservation measures mean that our homes are less draughty than they used to be, making them warmer and cosier for the mite. Some experts believe that as the fashion for fitted carpets has spread so have attacks of allergic asthma. Soft furnishings, too, provide an ideal environment, with an average home giving plenty of choice – lots of full curtains, frilly blinds and cosy, comfy sofas. Many of us sleep on mattresses which are several years old. Just think how much skin and perspiration they must have absorbed in that time, given that we spend an average of eight hours a night in bed. It has been estimated that up to ten per cent of the weight of an old pillow may be due to the mites – both live and dead ones – and their droppings. Again, not a very nice thought.

Mattresses should be thoroughly vacuumed and duvets or blankets taken to the dry cleaners. And we should consider having the bedroom carpets and curtains steam-cleaned, too. As we shed most of our microscopically small skin flakes in the bedroom, it's most important that we remove all the dust traps, as well as the dust.

Sometimes feathers can provoke an allergic response in the vulnerable. This again is probably due to the dust mite and to the 'dander' – the microscopic particles of feather – that can filter through the pillow case. Dust can more readily collect in feather than foam pillows, carrying the mites and their droppings with it. Covers which can be 'wet wiped' but which also allow air in and out of the pillow (so that they are not sweaty to lie on) are now available. These act like a filter, keeping the dander and the dust mites inside.

POLLUTION

Increasingly, specialists say that pollution does play a part in bringing on asthma attacks. Certainly, pollution can't be good, especially for anyone with asthma or a lung condition.

The main culprit in air pollution is sulphur-dioxide, which is released mainly by power stations burning coal. Car and lorry exhaust produces nitrogen-dioxide. Some people blame the increase in asthma on the rise in air pollution such as 'acid air' caused when car exhaust and other emissions containing sulphur-dioxide and nitrogen-oxides are released into the atmosphere. Even low levels of acid air can trigger asthma in those susceptible.

A more visible problem and one that hot sunny summers produce is the rise in pavement ozone level. Sunlight causes air pollutants to react and make ozone. Ozone, which forms a layer in the upper atmosphere, protects us from the sun's ultra-violet rays, yet when ozone is at ground level it can be harmful to lungs. Ozone helps form what is known as 'photochemical smog' with which I'm sure readers living in cities such as London and Manchester will be familiar after recent hot summers. Children are particularly sensitive to ozone which aggravates inflamed airways and makes allergies worse.

Tobacco smoke is the main indoor pollutant (see also page 48).

As already mentioned, the theory is that as the air we breathe becomes more polluted through industry and the motor car, air pollutants make the lungs more vulnerable to allergens such as pollens and viruses. Nitrogen-dioxide is particularly thought to add to your chances of picking up a virus infection such as flu, which in turn could trigger asthma attacks. According to the National Asthma Campaign, exhaust fumes, one of the main pollutants, have increased by seventy-five per cent since 1980. The situation isn't likely to improve either, because although some cars have catalytic converters many older cars do not, coupled with the fact that traffic volume could easily more than double within the next thirty years.

People often ask me whether living in a big city can give their child asthma. My own area of medical responsibility at one stage in my career covered a city-sized town as well as the green and leafy areas around it in Surrey. I studied the asthma cases being admitted to the local hospital – which therefore could be assumed to be the most severe – and discovered that more were being admitted from the green outer suburbs where the average household incomes were higher, than from the traffic-polluted city centre where the average household incomes were a lot smaller. This was occurring in the winter as well as the summer so pollen out of town was not the culprit. Closer examination suggested that the parents in the more affluent places in the country also had their own transport and were perhaps more assertive about what medical attention they needed when they saw symptoms starting, so they went straight to the hospital. However, such studies can only give a hint about what might be the real reason for our observations about the patterns of a medical condition.

Also, according to a recent *Evening Standard* article, one survey recently found that the incidence of asthma was as bad in Skye as it was in the centre of Aberdeen. It has also been suggested that ozone levels are probably higher in the country than cities because in the city ozone reacts again with some of the known causes of pollution and possibly has a partial neutralising effect – but we don't really know.

So pollution and asthma cause furious debate. Some believe that pollution itself causes asthma in people who have never suffered from it before, while others argue that it only triggers asthma in those susceptible. The other problem when looking at pollution is that asthma is a very individual thing. Asthmatics are all different, they react differently to different triggers, for example; they have the condition to varying degrees and have different levels of treatment, so it is hard to apply one theory to cover every case. The problem is that while pollutants such as nitrogen-dioxide, particularly when combined with sulphur-dioxide, can make asthma worse for a sufferer, some experts argue they don't actually cause asthma in the first place.

But if you feel air pollution triggers your asthma you can listen out for air quality warnings on weather forecasts or ring the Department of the Environment's Air Quality Information Line on 0800 556677, which gives summaries of air quality across the country as well as individual readings for nitrogen-dioxide (our main town pollutant), sulphur-dioxide (an urban and rural pollutant coming from industry) and ground level ozone. When air quality is poor or very poor, you may find that your breathing is not as easy as normal if you have asthma or bronchitis.

In the old 'pea soup' fogs experienced especially in London but also in Britain's other cities before the clean air acts became law, at the time of each fog the numbers of people admitted to hospital and dying from chest troubles would rise alarmingly. In fact it was as a result of the large number of deaths caused by one such pea-souper in the early 1950s that it was decided by Parliament that something had to be done. I have no doubt that fog has a seriously detrimental effect upon the symptoms of most people's asthma.

Very good air quality means that there is not much air pollution around. Poor or very poor air means there is a lot of air pollution around. Air quality tends to get worse on calm still days when there is no wind to blow the pollution away.

If air quality warnings are bad you should seek the advice of your GP or practice nurse about how you should deal with air pollution of this nature. GPs sometimes advise patients to double their inhaled preventive treatment or, if already using it twice a day, they may suggest that it may be useful to add a dose in the middle of the day, since the concentration of ozone in the atmosphere peaks in the afternoon. Or if suffering from mild asthma and no preventative medicine is used, it may be prescribed until the air quality improves. Some patients may need to travel by car or bus, rather than walking when air quality is very poor.

What else can you do? Those whose asthma is related to pollen may even need to stay indoors with windows and doors shut when the pollen counts are announced as being particularly high – at least in the morning and evening when the pollen is rising as the heat of the day carries it up and vice versa at the end of the day when it is descending. You might prefer to avoid outdoor strenuous exercise when air quality is poor.

Many people suffering from asthma have asked me when something is likely to be done about the harm to the environment caused by pressurised aerosol inhalers, also known as metered dose inhalers (MDIs). They are concerned about the effect on the ozone layer from pollution, though at the same time 'adding' to that pollution because of their inhalers.

The active drug in the inhaler is suspended in a propellant which forms a spray when the inhaler is pressed. Until now the propellants used have been chlorofluorocarbons (CFCs), substances which contribute to the destruction of the ozone layer, the protective mantle between the earth's surface and the sun, which limits the amount of ultraviolet (UV) radiation reaching the earth's surface.

While the use of CFCs in other areas – in hairsprays and deodorants, for instance – has declined, metered dose inhalers are one of the last sources of CFCs escaping into the atmosphere. Fortunately, one has recently been marketed which is, at long last, environmentally friendly. This is just as well since between 440 and 500 million metered dose inhalers are used world-wide and some experts believe that by the year 2000 it could be as many as 800 million.

Depletion of the ozone layer provokes public interest because it could signify increasing levels of harmful UV radiation reaching the earth's surface, which can cause skin cancers, cataracts and other eye problems, as well as damage to the human immune system, reducing our capacity to fight disease and infection.

Under the terms of the Montreal Protocol on Substances that Deplete the Ozone Layer, the manufacture of CFCs was banned in Europe from January 1995. However, inhalers for asthma were given a temporary exemption from this ban. As well as the fact that millions of asthma sufferers rely on these inhalers, time was needed to develop and test a substitute propellant. 3M Health Care's new inhaler contains HFA-134a, a propellant which does not cause destruction of the ozone layer. It has taken five years for 3M Health Care to produce this new CFC-free metered dose inhaler to deliver salbutamol, the most commonly used medication to relieve asthma symptoms. The new product is called the Airomir salbutamol sulphate CFC-free metered dose inhaler.

I welcome its introduction. And Frank Ellis, managing director of 3M Health Care says, 'The introduction of the CFC-free metered dose inhaler is particularly significant as asthma and the use of inhalers is increasing in the Western World.'

For seventy-five-year-old Allan, who first developed asthma when he was sixty, there is no shadow of a doubt that the rise in the incidence of asthma is linked to pollution.

> When you first get asthma you certainly are very scared. Not being able to breathe was something I had never come across before. I was surprised, as I had never been ill before in my life.
>
> I now feel quite angry about pollution. It's very bad here in Hull because we are practically below sea-level and our main pollution problem is lorries. We have many going through Hull centre. We have bypasses but lorry drivers seem to want to take the shortest route. In summer time when it's muggy and there is a bit of hazy sunshine it really is terrible.
>
> I know that I would start with a semi-attack with tightness in the chest and restricted breathing if I went into the town at this time. Pollution of this nature affects all asthmatics. Two thousand die every year and pollution must play a part in this. You see, everybody ignores pollution: councillors, county councillors, MPs – they all fight shy of pollution because they say traffic restrictions affect trade. But other countries don't allow traffic in the centre of their towns.
>
> There is no doubt in my mind that the increase in pollution is linked to the increase in asthma patients. I blame lorries and old cars. You can sit in any street and watch old cars go by and some of them are burning more oil than petrol and the fumes that come out of

exhausts are disgusting. Some buses are the same.

There should be more restrictions on traffic or restrictions at different times of the day. Deliveries could be made early on in the day so that for the rest of the day towns are traffic free. It's not an impossible situation. It only needs a few people with common sense to devise a route for deliveries to get rid of this excessive pollution.

ASTHMA AND EXERCISE

Exercise is a common asthma trigger. Some people suffer from exercise-induced asthma, also called exercise asthma, which means symptoms of asthma are brought on by exercise. For some sufferers exercise-induced asthma may occur in isolation, or it can be but one of several of their triggers.

Running in cold weather or undertaking sporting activities when pollen levels are high or when you've just got over a cold, are times when exercise can cause an asthma attack. Research scientists observe what's happening in a sufferer's tissues by looking at the response produced by the mast cells. These cells are responsible for releasing histamine and several other similar chemicals which cause many of the symptoms of both allergies and asthma. They can see the mast cells change as they lose a granular – grain-like – appearance within their substance, when seen under a microscope. This 'degranulation' gives the scientists a measure of an individual's tissue response to the trigger, and consequently they observe this closely.

Scientists can also observe how successfully the symptoms can be relieved by sodium cromoglycate (Intal). It is likely that the mast cell's response, and therefore the tissue response, to exercise is caused by the increased rush of air taken in and exhaled during exercise abrading the unduly sensitive tissues of a sufferer and so triggering the asthma symptoms.

So how can you tell when wheezing means the start of an asthma attack or a shortness of breath that normally follows exertion? Well, although breathlessness is common after strenuous exercise, even in an athlete, wheezing is not. And if the breathlessness doesn't recover in about a minute or you find it quite impossible to speak at the same time, it is a good enough reason for consulting your doctor.

With correct treatment exercise-induced asthma can be well controlled. Sufferers should not avoid sport and exercise as in general the long-term benefits outweigh any short-term risks. If you have asthma you should try to take exercise, but not to the point of exhaustion. You can enjoy most sports and prevent an asthma attack by taking two puffs of a bronchodilator inhaler fifteen minutes before starting.

Samantha, a twenty-one-year-old temporary clerical worker who has had asthma from childhood, has found that swimming has been an enjoyable form of exercise and one which helps keep her fit. She believes you shouldn't avoid exercise just because you have asthma and it's a matter of finding the right type of exercise to suit you.

> I was diagnosed as having asthma when I was about four but I had had lots of coughs before that age. I can remember having the

first asthma attack when I was about six. From that age until around ten I had a bad spell of attacks. I went to an asthma clinic every Tuesday which involved learning how to breathe and how to keep control in an attack and how parents could help. I also used to go to a swimming club which was run by the clinic on a Saturday morning in order to help me breathe better. And I think it did help me at the time.

Asthma wasn't as frightening for me as you might imagine it would be for a child. I was aware at the time of an attack of feeling frightened because when you have a tight chest you feel as if you are suffocating. I didn't think I was going to die or anything because I had had it from such an early age it was part of me. It wasn't like suddenly having an attack one day when you have never had one before. It was just something that I always had. I didn't feel isolated. I wasn't even the only one in my class with asthma. There were three of us in our class and one of them was my friend. So I didn't feel particularly different from other children. It didn't really bother me. It only restricted PE or running sometimes when it was cold but I still did games when I could.

I don't get attacks very often now I'm older. Between the ages of seven and fourteen was my worst time. I missed school but not enough to make a difference. I usually get asthma if I have a cold or if I am upset about things – if I'm holding things in or stressed about things. I remember when I was young while my asthma was bad I was

> being bullied at school. A few of us who were quiet were bullied by one particular girl. I can't remember what she used to say to us but I remember she used to pick on me and I would go home at night holding it all in. I went through a phase when I would not want the light off at night and I would cry. My parents couldn't understand why but eventually it all came out. My asthma was definitely worse then because of my emotions.
>
> When my grandparents died it affected my chest. Around my exams it does get a little worse. It didn't bring on an attack but I did feel a tightness at night.

Samantha still has asthma now, but the attacks are not as frequent as they were in her childhood.

> Looking back at my attacks, they are clearly linked with stressful situations or if I have a cold. Cats also affect me.
>
> When I was younger I used to get a lot of backache because of asthma at the top of my back and in the small of my back. I think it might have been the way I would hold myself tense when I knew an attack was coming on. I'd also get an itchiness around my chin or I would feel itchy and tickly inside as an attack was coming on. It was almost as if I could sense an attack about to start. Then my chest would get tighter. Attacks would build up with a cough, then a tightness or a loose bark. My asthma never just comes on really suddenly.
>
> For instance, I remember one attack when

I was about eight when I was at a friend's and I stopped overnight. I coughed through the night and in the morning my chest got tighter and tighter. We called a doctor who told me to breathe through a bottle. We got an orange squash bottle and squeezed the inhaler into that. I was so short of breath I couldn't breathe in to get a full dose of medicine.

I used to have a preventer but now I just have Ventolin. It's very rare that I go anywhere without it. I feel better knowing that if I need it I've got it there. But I do find that other people panic more than I do, friends more than family, even if I just take my inhaler. I recently went to Spain on holiday with friends and my friends were smoking so I had to take my inhaler. Discos make my chest tight, the smoky atmosphere and especially the dry ice. I have to say don't worry, I'm fine. If I feel my symptoms coming on I will take my inhaler wherever I am. I just turn my back away from people slightly for a bit of privacy and to stop people asking me if I'm okay or wondering what is happening. Sometimes it's worse dealing with people who are asking you questions when you can't breathe properly than dealing with your asthma and trying to get your medication sorted out. If my chest feels really tight I will sit down and bend over slightly to ease my breathing.

I don't feel my parents were particularly over-protective. I was brought up normally. My grandfather had asthma too so it was just part of family life really. I know my mother would worry at night if she didn't hear my breathing or coughing. She wouldn't be able to sleep properly. I might have just dropped off to sleep and she would come in and check on me.

Asthma has disturbed my sleep with coughing. It gets worse at night – I either cough or if my chest is tight I can't lie down or I can't settle. I can't get comfortable. If I lie flat it's worse, so I sit up and you can't sleep like that. Or sometimes when I cough and it sounds like a loud bark I get anxious because I am disturbing everyone. There's no point everyone being up. I feel bad about keeping the family up at night when they have to go to work the next day as well. My asthma might not be so bad during the day but I feel so tired after a night like that.

You have to lead a normal life and get on with it. It's not worth worrying about but make sure you get good advice. That way you can learn to deal with asthma and know when to take your inhalers. You can't let asthma rule your life. You just get to know your own limitations and build your life around that. Even now I can't run or I can't do a lot of aerobics but that doesn't put me off doing exercise. After a while I have to stop because I can feel my chest becoming tight. When this happens I either go slowly or stop and take my inhaler, or if it carries on I drop out altogether.

I can't do an hour of aerobics but I don't get upset about it, I just go swimming instead. There are top athletes who are asthmatics and their condition hasn't stopped them achieving things. Obviously there are people who have asthma worse than I have it but a lot of people can carry on as near normal as possible. There's no point sitting around bemoaning the fact that you have asthma.

ASTHMA, STRESS AND EMOTIONS

Asthma is a condition with a clear link to stress. Many different stressors can cause an attack, even a heavy meal which may have a stressful effect on the body.

We're most likely to become sick in our body's weak spot. If we have a weak spot in our throat, then that could be where stress would affect us. So if our chest is our weak spot stressful situations or being under stress without realising it could result in an attack.

Stress to one person may not be stress to another. As some sufferers have told me, they're not even aware they are under stress until their asthma symptoms worsen. Of course, it is not always possible to remove stress factors from your life as it affects us all every day. And from all the calls I receive on the *Jimmy Young Show*, as well as letters I'm sent regularly, I've reached the conclusion that recognising that we're stressed, why we should be so and then acting to solve the problem isn't easy for anyone. It can be hard for many people just to admit that they feel stressed – so often they feel it is viewed as a sign of weakness, or of not being able to do their job properly, or a confession that they are in fact feeling very lonely.

However, stress isn't always a bad thing. Positive stress, or pressure, is needed for us to work well and to drive us to get the most out of life.

Your personality and just the way you're made can decide how much stress you can take – but that doesn't mean to say that asthma sufferers can't tolerate pressure or are made in a different way to everybody else. As with all forms of stress, particularly emotional stress, if you can find ways of dealing with or reducing your stress it is highly likely that the frequency and severity of your asthma will be reduced as well.

Stress alone won't cause asthma, but if you do suffer from asthma it can bring on an attack or make your day-to-day symptoms worse. Audrey, a fifty-seven-year-old housewife, has recently been told she's suffering from asthma which is likely to be stress-induced. Her symptoms, a constant cough, became much more evident following the unexpected and tragic death of her husband three years ago. It seems the grief and emotional trauma she has experienced has triggered her symptoms.

> I think I might have had asthma before my husband's death. Looking back to about six months before he died, I can remember bouts of coughing. I have never smoked but my husband did smoke. If I came into the kitchen in the morning and he had been smoking I would start to cough and would have to open the windows. Coming into contact with cigarette smoke definitely affected my coughing.
>
> Then three years ago my husband passed away. He had a massive heart attack at the age of fifty-three and he died in front of me.

He hadn't shown signs of any suffering before then. I think the shock of seeing him die is still with me. Then it was hard to adjust to a single life and having to do everything for myself again. It seemed that within a few months I started coughing, and have been coughing ever since. It's not bad enough to keep me awake at night but it's always there. I've also had continuous colds and felt under the weather – which could also be part of the grief. I didn't experience any wheezing, I just sounded full of cold all the time and I couldn't stop coughing. As soon as I woke in the morning I would cough, if the temperature changed I would cough – if I went out from a warm room into cold air, or if I climbed upstairs in the house. I walk a lot and that didn't seem to affect my cough, but I found that if I had to walk upstairs in a car park it did make my cough worse.

Initially my doctor didn't say it was asthma, he just told me it was all part of the grief. But a couple of months ago I had a terrible bout of flu and I was in bed for ten days. That was when my doctor told me he thought I might have asthma and as soon as I was well enough I should come to the surgery.

When I did see him again I had to blow into a peak flow meter and he told me that the reading was very low for someone of my age. He gave me a steroid inhaler, Pulmicort, to take four times a day to see how my symptoms responded. I have been taking it for a month and I do feel better and my voice is much clearer. And all my family and friends tell me so as well. I really do feel a lot different.

My doctor thinks I have chronic asthma and that my air tubes are inflamed. He advised me in a couple of weeks to cut down on my inhaler to twice a day. But he warned me that this is likely to be always with me to a certain extent, particularly in the winter time, or if I have a cold. To be told I have asthma came as quite a shock to me, I always thought someone with asthma would have far worse symptoms than I have.

ASTHMA AND SMOKING

Many sufferers tell me that as well as causing other allergic reactions such as irritated eyes, runny noses or even sore throats, cigarette smoke can trigger an asthma attack. It is not surprising that this should be so as cigarette smoke causes a mild though chronic (continuous) inflammation of the lining of the nose, throat and lung airways. This makes the now 'roughened' surface far more likely to pick up any passing infection or any passing allergen. The British Allergy Foundation points out that cigarette smoke has indeed been reported to increase the risks of allergy in some people. In someone who already has an allergic type of eczema, cigarette smoke is even more likely to provoke asthmatic problems.

Cigarettes are thought to be one of the worst pollutants we can come across, containing hydrocarbons, carbon-monoxide, nicotine and nitrogen-dioxide, and they are a great problem for non-smokers because the smoke is difficult to avoid as only about a quarter is inhaled by the smoker.

If you suffer from asthma and you smoke you should try to stop smoking. It is thought that every year some 100,000 people in the UK die because of smoking-related problems. These problems are mainly lung cancer, chronic obstructive lung disease (often previously known as chronic bronchitis) or coronary heart disease. Every day around 300 Britons die as a direct result of smoking. Each time you light up, just think about those 4000 substances in cigarette smoke (the majority poisonous) that you are inhaling.

People often tell me that they don't believe there's much point in giving up smoking because they've smoked for so many years that the damage has been done. Well, that's not true. As soon as you give up smoking your lungs begin to return to normal. Within eight hours the levels of nicotine and carbon-monoxide in your blood will have decreased by fifty per cent just for a start – and it gets better with each hour and the longer term benefits with every day. So it really is worth a try.

There are many new aids on the market for giving up smoking. Your pharmacist can give you advice on these products, but only you can give up cigarettes. Determination is what is most needed. Studies have shown that seven out of ten smokers are likely to have tried to stop smoking and have subsequently failed. Don't be frightened to ask the help of your GP. Make a list of your reasons for wanting to stop. The list should include the facts that you'll run the risk of fewer asthma attacks, you'll be fitter, have fresher smelling clothes and hair, and a sense of achievement if you succeed, and just think of all the money you'll save! You may also consider trying a 'Stop Smoking' therapist, listening to an audio tape on the subject, or trying acupuncture or hypnotherapy. Enquire at your local library for services near you.

You don't have to smoke yourself in order to have your health endangered. Passive smoking is just as bad an irritant to an asthma sufferer. People still ask me what is meant by passive smoking. Passive smoking means breathing other people's tobacco smoke. You'll find tobacco smoke around whenever a cigarette, pipe or cigar is smoked, which could be in homes, public places or even at work for some people. It is considered as a major pollutant. The smoke that is purposely inhaled by the smoker is referred to as the main-stream smoke. The smoke that leads to the passive smoking is called side-stream smoke. It comes straight from the point of burning. It is this side-stream smoke which comes from the burning point of the tobacco itself, rather than the smoke which is consumed or inhaled by the smoker and subsequently puffed out, that is the major addition to the smoke in a room.

Passive smoking does pose a serious threat to children. There is evidence that children frequently exposed to tobacco smoke, for instance those whose parents are smokers, are more prone to respiratory infections and symptoms such as wheezing. Passive smoking may also contribute to chronic middle-ear disease in children. This is because smoking irritates and thus inflames the lining membranes in the breathing tubes including those – the Eustachian tubes – that connect the back of the nose to the middle ear to equalise the pressures behind the ear-drum. The inflammation causes swelling which can block those tubes, causing secretions to collect in the middle ear, making infection much more likely.

There is some indication that women who are heavily exposed to tobacco smoke during pregnancy may have lower-birth-weight babies. Women who smoke while they are pregnant actually increase the likelihood of their child being born with breathing difficulties or developing asthma. There's also a theory that the more cigarette smoke you are exposed to as a child the more likely you are to develop respiratory disease when you are an adult. Passive smoking has been shown to have a severe and damaging effect on those with existing respiratory conditions such as asthma.

Elizabeth, a fifty-nine-year-old nurse, has suffered with asthma since she was a child. She is able to manage it efficiently by daily medication and conscientious use of a peak flow meter. She has refused to let it over-rule her life but she does resent having to think about whether or not people will be smoking if she's going out socially and tries to avoid cigarette smoke wherever she can.

'When I was young you didn't have asthma as such and you were regarded as a child with a wheezy chest.'

Throughout her twenties her asthma began to get worse and she believes she could have sought better treatment earlier than she did. Elizabeth believes that if you have asthma you should face up to it and seek medical help and advice. Don't just ignore it and hope it will go away.

> Go to your doctor or asthma clinic and do take their advice. Asthma can turn very

dramatically. If you have a cold or chest infection, do check it out with your doctor. They can be just bad enough to trigger your asthma problems. Always seek your doctor's advice about asthma. Most doctors are very asthma aware these days.

I use a peak flow meter every day and it really is a useful guide to your ability to breathe out air. If you have been assessed you will know what your usual marker will be, depending on your age, height and sex. Each person's regime is different and you know if you go below a certain level what course of action to take.

Using a peak flow is part of my life. I use it when I get up in the morning. Ideally you should do it before your medication and then about an hour or so later take another reading. I don't always have time if I'm rushing off to work to do a post peak flow reading. If I am late for work sometimes I take the meter with me and do the reading at work when I can. You can keep a diary of your peak flow readings. They are useful because you can see whether you are improving or going down.

When you have an asthma attack breathing out quickly becomes very difficult. It's more difficult to breathe out than breathe in although neither is easy. I used to get in a panic now and then but I think my nurse's training must have helped me and I also used to do yoga.

Yoga was helpful to me at times when I was aware early enough that my chest was becoming tight; I tried to relax and take slow, gentle breaths. One of the frustrating things about asthma is that you always have to remember to take your inhaler with you even if you are just going down to the local shop. And if I have done the unforgivable thing of going out without my inhalers – which unfortunately happened on one or two occasions – I would panic about it. So I would try to eliminate the panic from my thoughts and reassure myself that I had done all my treatments before I came out. Then I would try to breathe slowly and carefully as I had been taught in yoga. That did work for me. I'm not saying yoga is the answer – you still need medication for asthma. But relaxing through yoga techniques can help you if you are going into a panic.

But, that said, I haven't allowed asthma to restrict my life. I used to do cycle racing. Now I am older my lifestyle has changed and I don't cycle as much as I used to because I do notice air pollution more now, especially caused by the London traffic, particularly when it's hot. I don't go up to London if I have a choice. But if the atmosphere is heavy or the air is very cold it can close down the airways and at these times I am very aware of my breathing.

Elizabeth sometimes gets fed up about not being able to do 'horse duties' for the St John Ambulance because being in contact with horses, say at the Windsor Horse Show, or Royal Ascot, will affect her chest. When talking about living with asthma, one of the issues which makes Elizabeth extremely angry is cigarette smoking in public places. This is a particular problem for her in restaurants and pubs. She is conscious that many smokers underestimate the impact of their smoking on asthma sufferers and certainly, she feels, do not realise that, for many asthma sufferers, cigarette smoke alone can trigger an attack. She is also resentful about the restrictions that the presence of cigarette smoke imposes on her social life.

> Asthma tends to restrict my social life most of all. I don't have a very hectic social life and I don't stop going out to dinner. But if I am going to an organised dinner I do state I want to be in a non-smoking area and if there won't be one, I won't go. I always ask for no-smoking areas when we go to restaurants. I just wish more restaurants had them. I have no problems with cinemas now since smoking has been banned. Most of my friends don't smoke so that doesn't pose me any extra problems. I will not go to a pub. I will not go anywhere where there is likely to be smoking and I do resent this restriction.

POLLEN

Pollen causes problems for many people with or without asthma. Some people suffer from hay-fever and about one in ten sufferers find that pollen can be an allergy trigger factor for their asthma, sparking off symptoms such as coughing, chest tightness and wheezing. If you wheeze with your hay-fever it is likely to mean that it is causing asthma symptoms for you.

Hayfever is an allergic reaction which occurs in people who are particularly sensitive to pollen or spores released into the air by trees, grasses or moulds. Its medical name is seasonal allergic rhinitis and it is now one of the most common allergies known. It is estimated that between six and twelve million people suffer – mostly between the ages of ten and forty, with about one in six teenagers affected. It is also estimated that four million working days are lost during June and July alone through hayfever.

Hayfever strictly refers to an allergy to grass pollen, but the term is often used to cover allergy to pollen from plants, shrubs and trees. People suffering from asthma can also be allergic to the many types of pollen we unavoidably come into contact with. Pollens released in spring are usually from trees, while in the summer flower, grass or weed pollens are released. In the autumn the symptoms are usually caused by pollen from autumn-flowering plants and the spores of some fungi. The symptoms experienced are due not to the pollen itself, but to the body's reaction to it. The sufferer's body reacts to pollen as though it were a potentially dangerous threat such as a germ, which is why some people suffering from hayfever for the first time think it is the onset of a heavy cold with a congested nose, running eyes and maybe also a wheeze as it has 'gone to the chest'. In fact some of the changes seen with all types of asthma are due to inflammation, similar to those seen with a chest infection. The inflammation causes a swelling of the lining membrane of the breathing tubes in the same way that inflammation caused by an infection causes an inflammation of the breathing tubes.

During a hay-fever attack, catechol amines (around twenty different chemicals, including histamine) are released from the mast cells in the tissues. These amines attract the white blood cells (platelets), which are part of the body's defence mechanism to fight infection and which are known to be associated with inflammation. The ones mainly attracted are the eosinophils, so called because they can be stained with eosin to stand out from the others when viewed under a microscope.

Again, the concentration of these cells sets up a damaging inflammatory reaction, similar to that which would deal with a dangerous germ invasion. In the case of hay-fever, however, the sufferer has to put up with the 'battle' which was not necessary in the first place, for the pollen would not otherwise have caused harm – as is the case with those who don't suffer even though they are still subject to the same pollen.

The eyes water in an effort to wash away the pollen and the running nose and sneezing help to eject the 'invader'. Virtually all sufferers get nasal symptoms, eight out of ten eye symptoms, and as many as six out of ten may get some 'pollen' wheezing as well. Of this last group, the misery of the symptoms can, rarely, be overshadowed by the threat of a more serious acute asthmatic attack requiring hospital treatment for its relief.

Hay-fever sufferers and those whose asthma is aggravated by pollen are most at risk between May and September, when the pollen count (the level of pollen in the air) is at its highest. So listen to the pollen count forecasts broadcast daily on television and local radio or check the weather reports in newspapers. A pollen count of fifty grains per cubic metre is enough to set most sufferers sneezing. The pollen count will be high on warm, dry and windy days because pollen released from grasses and trees is carried upwards by warm air. Also, warm, dry conditions are needed for pollen to be released in the first place.

Symptoms are often more severe in the morning, when pollen is released and carried upwards as the air temperature rises. They then become worse again in the evening as the temperature drops and the pollen grains drift back down. There is a growing body of medical evidence which points to a new link between pollution and hay-fever. Studies show that pollution has an adjuvant effect on pollen, enhancing sensitisation and in some cases actually sensitising atopic individuals to airborne allergens. (Atopic individuals are those who may already be more susceptible because of an increased level of a certain antibody in their blood which they will have inherited from one or both of their parents.)

Hay-fever can be treated effectively and you should seek the advice of your doctor or pharmacist. Some people who have asthma but who also react to pollen may need additional medication during the hay-fever season for their asthma, as well as preparations for their nasal and eye symptoms.

If you suffer from hay-fever and/or asthma which is triggered by pollen you can try to minimise your exposure. Wearing plain glasses or sunglasses can prevent much of the eye irritation, by stopping pollen grains entering the eyes. Avoid walking through grass or cutting it. Keep windows and doors closed, especially when lawns are being mowed. Stay away from pets if they have been outside. Try to plan your day to avoid being outdoors in the morning and evening when pollen counts are at their highest. Don't go on country walks and avoid parks or gardens on warm and sunny days, or, if this is impossible, wash your hair afterwards. Keep car windows and air vents closed when you're out driving.

ASTHMA AND INFECTIONS

Chest infections such as the common cold or bronchitis are very common triggers for asthma for adults as well as children (see also page 6). It is almost as if the narrowing of the breathing tubes which an infection can cause, as the lining membrane swells to fight the infection, triggers the full asthmatic response – which includes a muscle contraction of the tubes themselves, making the breathing passages even narrower as their muscles contract.

And the reverse is also likely to occur. Because of the narrowing of the breathing tubes, as well as the swelling of their lining, both of which are present in asthma, chest infections are also more likely to be able to take hold during an asthma attack.

ASTHMA AND OTHER MEDICINES

Should people with asthma avoid certain medicines, I am often asked. If you have asthma you shouldn't worry unduly about taking other medicines generally, but there are some specific medicines it is best to avoid as they could cause problems for some asthmatics.

About one in fifty asthmatics is allergic to aspirin so it's probably best to avoid – unless advised otherwise by your doctor – taking aspirin or products containing or relating to aspirin (such as certain drugs for arthritis) particularly as paracetamol is a safe alternative.

Asthma sufferers and anyone who is allergic to aspirin should only take ibuprofen after consulting their doctor. Ibuprofen, also known commonly by one of its brand names, Nurofen, is an NSAID (non-steroidal anti-inflammatory drug) which relieves pain, reduces inflammation and lowers temperature. It does this, in common with other NSAIDs, by reacting against the body's locally released chemical responsible for those symptoms – the prostaglandins.

Asthmatics should also avoid another group of drugs, known as beta-blockers, which are commonly used to treat angina and high blood pressure and act on the nerves which control circulation. Beta-blockers can also be prescribed to patients under great stress. For someone with a tendency to asthma beta-blockers can provoke an attack.

Always remind your doctor, or mention to your pharmacist if you are thinking of buying an over-the-counter medicine, that you have asthma so that you can be offered safe alternatives that won't affect your asthma.

HOW TO DEAL WITH YOUR DOCTOR

Asthma is one of the most common conditions – if not the most common – that GPs come across in their surgeries, and it is one that is spread right across the age range.

Control of your asthma does not fall mainly on your doctor. You have to take control too. Do talk to your doctor about aspects of your asthma which may not seem important to you in the strict medical sense or which you may have come to accept as your lot. Waking up at night because of your asthma, for example, deserves a mention to your doctor. Far too many sufferers accept this as normal. Nocturnal waking can be a sign that asthma is becoming worse or that you may need more treatment. You shouldn't just put up with it as it can also mean that you're functioning generally less well because you become over-tired and irritable during the day. A drug such as salmeterol (Serevent) may be prescribed. This is a fairly new drug and is called a protector as its effects last for around twelve hours. It works by keeping the lung's air passages open and relaxed in order to facilitate breathing. A protector is usually prescribed for use in conjunction with a preventer, such as an inhaled steroid.

Your GP and practice nurse will be involved with the management of your asthma. Many GP practices, especially the larger ones, now hold special asthma clinics, as they may also do for other groups of conditions which need regular medical monitoring, such as diabetes. This is a very helpful change in the way practices have been reorganised over recent years. Many practice nurses, in particular, have obtained further training in asthma management and have become specialists with particular expertise in the day-to-day care and advice that is needed by sufferers. Delia, a forty-two-year-old National Asthma Centre training instructor, believes strongly in the new approach of well-informed asthma management to overcome the different perceptions of asthma in different age groups and cultures.

> I suppose everybody has an underlying fear of what it would be like if they had a bad attack. But people with asthma don't tend to say that upfront. It depends very much too on what age group you are talking about.
>
> People of my age have a different perspective on what asthma means to, say, a child these days – because it's so common now. When I was at school very few people had asthma diagnosed. And the ones who were diagnosed as having asthma were diagnosed because it couldn't possibly be anything else. It was glaringly obvious. In the 1960s it was still considered that there was an element of it all being in their head. There weren't the inhaled steroids available and treatment often consisted of just bronchodilators or people were put straight on to oral steroids. Consequently they had the side-effects often associated with oral steroids. Because of that there was the taboo of labelling someone as asthmatic. It was a vicious circle.

So if somebody asked me who I knew from my childhood with asthma I could think of two people who perhaps were very bad. Carrying that thought further, if I didn't know anything about asthma and went to my doctor to be told my child had asthma I might be more panicky than someone who has only known about asthma as it is now – when more people seem to have it than not.

I have my own personal theory about the increase in asthma. It occurred to me that we all wear man-made fibres a lot now. I don't say they give off fumes but they could lose very fine particles and we could be inhaling them all the time. When you think of how you can be allergic to something like a washing powder, maybe this is a factor – combined with all the other factors such as house dust mites. I don't know so much about air pollution. There is quite a lot of controversy about that and I don't think it's a straightforward issue. If you have a child being pushed along in a buggy up a busy town high street at the level of exhaust pipes it probably contributes to their asthma. Researchers have tried to prove that it is a causative thing but all they have been able to come up with is that it is a catalyst. Air pollution is not going to cause asthma but if you have it it could make it worse.

I think the cause is a concoction of different things. There are so many different factors. For example, some people find if they move from one area to another, they either become asthmatic or they will get better in a different area.

> Other people talk about junk food and lack of exercise. But I have noticed when I question people about whether exercise brings on their asthma it seems that if they don't take much exercise and they suddenly run it will bring on their asthma. If they take regular exercise people often tell me that if they stop exercising their asthma gets worse.
>
> I also feel some people have problems with their nose. They have ENT problems, such as allergic rhinitis, and if that can be sorted out asthma often improves.
>
> Yet I don't think anybody is going to come up with an answer and say x equals asthma. I think the cause is a concoction of different things.

Asthma awareness has improved. Delia believes asthma clinics offer a useful service and that if they are on offer in your area you should make use of them.

> I think they have arisen in tandem with the increase in asthma. It's one of the few areas where you can prevent things happening by just informing people of what to do. People are definitely not as well informed about asthma as they should be. There are still a terrific number of people who are putting up with symptoms because they think it's part of their normal condition. Coughing at night, for instance. Or if you get an older person they'll tell you they get breathless going up a flight of stairs but they think that's a natural part of getting old. Asthma is

> something people seem to adjust to very much. Even if you get them better you still have to keep reinforcing the message about prevention and taking medication, otherwise they can slip back again.

There are other areas in asthma management that people should be made aware of, such as the things we have discussed earlier in the book, about how to cope in an attack, for instance.

> In East Berkshire, we are currently working on the production of an emergency treatment card. Somebody who is just on a reliever inhaler very occasionally can still suddenly come up against something that will give them an acute attack. If perhaps they had a card like this in a handbag or wallet they could look at it because they might have forgotten what they are supposed to do. The card will probably have their name and their doctor's name and phone number; their best peak flow reading, what sort of treatment they're on, what to do in a moderately severe attack and what to do in a severe attack. The other way of using it is at casualty. If when they get there, they can't talk, staff can quickly look at this card.

Being shown correct inhaler technique is also another aspect of a patient being better informed. This is because many people find it difficult to use their inhaler in a way that ensures they breathe in the medication at the time they press the release mechanism. Consequently, the dose may not get to where it is intended, down into the lungs.

HOW TO DEAL WITH YOUR DOCTOR 65

> Asthma nurses can help with this. There are still people who think you can give someone a metered dose inhaler and they will automatically be able to use it or if they can't use it, the nurse can teach them. That's not fair. You have to find the most suitable device for each person. I don't think people should be encouraged, either, to say my friend's got such and such, so I want the same, if their inhaler is working very well for them and they know how to use it. A lot of people won't want anything different and this can be one of the problems an asthma nurse comes up against where you have someone whose technique is appalling. If they try another type of inhaler and their technique improves they will still state their preference for their old one. It's because that is what they are used to and they trust it. Because asthmatics rely on their medication so much, some are very resistant to change. Even if something only changes colour slightly, people go up the wall!

Apart from understanding as much about the condition as you can, Delia's advice to people, particularly parents of children with asthma, is not to panic and to keep the school informed.

> It's very important that the school is informed. Some children are on preventing inhalers as well as some children who are on relievers; teachers need to understand the differences. In primary schools teachers must be informed – if a child is really feeling

bad he or she will know they need their inhaler but sometimes a child will soldier on and not ask for it, or a child will think it's a novelty and ask for it all the time.

Schools have different policies about inhalers. A lot of teachers are doing their best for children with asthma but if parents are not happy about the school's policy, as when a school will not keep inhalers for a child, it needs to go to county level. Our local primary school has wooden boxes with flip-top lids labelled inhalers. All the class's inhalers are put in there and the children can go to use them whenever they need to.

It's also useful to find out how many of you have children with asthma. Find out how many in your child's class have it. If you are talking about five or more in a class, you are quite a strong pressure group if you get together.

But I do think as well you should encourage parents and sufferers not to panic about asthma. It is very common and because we are getting better at diagnosing it, usually these days people can get by with minimal symptoms. In the 1960s it wasn't like that.

PREVENTION AND SELF-HELP TREATMENT

As I have already pointed out, people with asthma have airways which have become over-sensitive. This means that they are red and sore or inflamed most of the time. This, in turn, means that because they are already 'irritated' it doesn't take them long to react to allergens such as animals, cigarette smoke, air pollution or cold air. When they do react like this, these airways become even narrower. So if you suffer from asthma and know what triggers an attack, do obviously try to avoid the trigger. Your doctor is likely to have told you to do some or all of the following:

Wage a Campaign Against Dust

Keep your house as free from dust as possible. The National Asthma Campaign points out that around sixty per cent of all school children with asthma are allergic to house dust mite droppings. Try to minimise problems by vacuuming floors and furnishings and damp-dusting frequently. Polished floorboards or lino are less of a mite trap than carpets. Make sure you empty your vacuum cleaner bags frequently. It is also helpful not to vacuum while the person suffering from asthma is in the same room.

Mites thrive in warmth, so keep the bedroom cool and well aired. Smaller objects, such as children's fluffy toys, can be put into the deep freeze every so often for about six hours – mites cannot survive at that temperature. Sunlight also kills off the mites.

It really is important to wash sheets, pillowcases and duvet covers at very high temperatures. Newer washing powders and liquids have meant that clothes can now be effectively washed at lower temperatures, but in the case of the house dust mite the water needs to be pretty hot to kill them all off. You may need to invest in bed linen made of natural, rather than man-made fibres, which can withstand the higher washing temperatures.

If you find that house dust mites aggravate your asthma there are many products you can buy such as mite-proof zip-up mattress, pillow and duvet covers. These use a system of interliners, made from a special fabric, for mattresses, duvets and pillows, or come ready-fitted to a range of beds and pillows and work by preventing contact with house dust mites, and their droppings, during sleep. Slumberland, the bed manufacturers, also have a range which incorporates this technology into mattresses and pillows, which are available from Slumberland retailers. Try using pillows filled with artificial fibres rather than feathers. Trials have shown that 'allergic exclusion' of this nature can reduce allergic symptoms.

Studies show that careful avoidance of the house dust mite can bring about a significant reduction in the symptoms of allergic airways disease. Ask your pharmacist for advice about other products, such as sprays, to reduce mites.

Keep Rooms Well Aired

At home you should keep rooms well aired and try to cut down on condensation wherever possible. If there are any areas of walls with mould growing scrub it away as soon as you notice it, since mould can release tiny particles similar to pollen which could be yet another allergen your body has to deal with.

Don't Leave Home Without Them
Always keep your drugs close at hand.

Take as Directed
Always take your anti-inflammatory inhalations as instructed. These will usually be steroids and they are remarkably effective at preventing an attack.

Work Out a List of Trigger Factors
It is not always easy for asthma sufferers to work out what triggers their asthma. For some people it will always remain a mystery. But others find that awareness of certain trigger factors which they can avoid cuts down on the risk of an attack.

Kinaird, a sixty-five-year-old pensioner, tries to lead as normal a life as possible with the help of asthma medicines and by avoiding the trigger factors he knows will provoke an attack. He also finds it helps him cope with his asthma because he feels as if he is playing a part in controlling it.

> I've suffered with asthma for about eight years and over the years I have worked out as many of my trigger factors as I possibly can. Of course, I do rely on medication to cope with my asthma but it gives me peace of mind to think that I can also try to do something about avoiding attacks myself.

Some trigger factors are quite obvious but for others Kinaird has had to use a process of trial and error.

> I know about the obvious one like virus infection such as colds and flu. It's impossible to avoid catching them completely but I do make sure I have a flu vaccination each October to cut down the risk of having flu. I also find that if I catch a cold it always seems to go straight to my chest. I make sure I see my GP regularly when I think I might have an infection so that I get antibiotics prescribed for me as soon as I might need them.
>
> Dogs and cats are definite trigger factors for me. Just the smell of dogs affects me. If I go into a house where there's a dog, even if the dog isn't around there are the remains of a doggy smell, my chest goes tight and I have to leave immediately. Once I might have been polite and tried to stay a little longer but now my health comes first. I used to worry too much about people thinking I was neurotic. Now that's their problem and anyway I can always ring the person up to explain afterwards, although most of my family and friends know and understand how important it is for me to avoid my trigger factors.
>
> I have worked out over the years that all sorts of dust and even wood smoke do it. Coal fires don't seem to affect me too much but if someone has a log fire I can't be in the same room. New carpets bother me, I suppose because they give off lots of fluff and tiny fibres of wool for a few weeks. Flowers

PREVENTION AND SELF-HELP TREATMENT 71

and plants are definite triggers. I've even managed to work out exactly which ones so that we don't have any in our garden. Geraniums and lupins are very bad for me. Tomato plants are another trigger. Freshly cut grass also makes me wheeze, so my wife always has to mow our lawn and she collects the grass trimmings up immediately and puts them into a sealed black plastic bag and into the dustbin quickly.

Houseplants are no longer allowed at home. One of my doctors said that he was fed up with telling his patients that they needed to get rid of their houseplants because they are one of the worst things people with chest problems can keep.

Central heating is another trigger, especially when the air becomes too warm and dusty. Gas fires and electric fires affect me – although electric ones are slightly better than gas ones.

House dust mites – I can't have feather pillows and duvets. I even take my own pillows with me wherever I go. I make sure our sheets are washed at very high temperatures. My wife hangs out our duvet on the washing line when the sun is shining to give it a good airing and also to kill off any mites. She also regularly turns and vacuums the mattress. Anywhere where dust is being created is a no-go area for me. My wife has to do the vacuuming. If I have to do it then I wear a mask.

Cigarette smoke and car fumes – we've recently moved house to a much quieter street much higher up a hill because the fumes can trigger an attack. I really do notice the difference in the air quality. Where I used to live was quite a busy street and some days when the weather was very cold and there was a lot of stationary traffic my chest would tighten even if I only walked the short distance to the local newsagent.

Having to avoid cigarette fumes does restrict my social life. I am always being asked to the pub by friends and I always refuse. The other day I relented. It was lunchtime, the pub was quiet and there was only one person smoking in there, in a far corner. I wish I hadn't gone because that night my chest felt very tight and I coughed all night long. I'm sure it was just that slight contact with cigarette smoke that made the difference to my chest and my night's sleep. It just wasn't worth it and the next day I was worn out.

Hot, spicy food is the worst. Any foods containing chilli or a lot of pepper also produce an allergic response in me, and I have difficulty breathing. Cold air and sea air irritate me too. Sometimes I get fed up always having to think about what triggers my asthma. Then other days I realise it is worthwhile because anything that helps you cut down your asthma symptoms has to be good.

Do What You've Been Told

If you feel your asthma is getting worryingly worse, you should follow your doctor's instructions – often now printed as treatment guidelines and given to sufferers or their carers as soon as the diagnosis has been made. But when in doubt, contact your doctor.

Be Prepared
A friend of mine who has a son with severe asthma always told him to retain two small coins in one particular pocket so that he could phone her from wherever he was when he knew a bad attack was coming on and she would collect him. It is as well she suggested two coins. When he first felt the need to phone, all his mother heard were very deep breaths – the poor little chap could not even get a word out. She thought he was a heavy breather and put the phone down on him, only realising as she did so who it was. Thankfully, he managed to get the next coin in and she went to his aid.

Be Informed About Air Quality
See page 100 for more about the Department of the Environment's Pollution line. Get advice about how your asthma can be controlled when air quality is bad.

Don't Smoke
You shouldn't smoke and you should also avoid passive smoking (see also page 50). It is especially important for children with asthma to avoid cigarette smoke and you should be strict about anyone smoking near your children, particularly visitors to your house. One survey highlighted the fact that as many as a quarter of people with asthma were smokers!

Try to Exercise

Even though exercise can bring on wheezing, moderate exercise, such as swimming, should be undertaken, especially by asthmatic children. Using a bronchodilator drug before exercise helps prevent an attack. The National Asthma Campaign advises that you should exercise outside on warmer days (unless pollution levels are high) and inside on cold ones.

Use a Peak Flow Meter

Many doctors suggest that the regular use of a peak flow meter can help sufferers or their carers measure the progress of the asthma. These are simple gauges which, when you blow as hard as you can into them, measure the peak expiratory flow, which is a very good indicator of how well the lungs are functioning. These meters can be prescribed on the NHS.

Your peak flow measurement will depend on your age, height and whether you are male or female. Men have a higher peak flow than women. Younger people tend to have higher readings than older ones.

If you are troubled by asthma attacks fairly often, using a peak flow meter may help you keep a check on your asthma or warn you when extra treatment or medical advice might be needed. A peak flow meter helps assess and monitor asthma. In asthma, because airways become narrow and sensitive, it is harder to breathe out than to breathe in. Consequently, when you breathe out you exhale a smaller quantity of air than when your airways are 'good' or than someone not troubled by asthma.

For most people it is not the actual reading that

is the essential guideline – what is important is that you should be aware of any changes between morning and night and how much it varies from day to day. Asthma is such a variable condition that you could have a good morning or a bad afternoon and that is why the variations in peak flow readings help you work out how narrow your airways are. Wide variations can indicate that your asthma is getting worse or that your medication needs to be better controlled.

Wrap Up!
Wear a scarf around your face on cold days. It's likely that this allows some of your expired warm air to warm up the scarf, which then warms the next in-suck of air.

Try Ionisers
You could try using domestic ionisers, which are small electrical appliances that stabilise the negative electrical charges of split atoms floating in the air. Proponents claim that these can 'cure' many symptoms, including perennial rhinitis, sore eyes, and even asthma. However, like most doctors, I'm sceptical.

GOING ON HOLIDAY

Don't forget that when you go on holiday you will need to take sufficient supplies with you to cover all eventualities. If you're thinking of going away you should ask your doctor or pharmacist for advice. You may need to ask him whether your particular medication and the way you use it will need to be handled differently in a hot country, for example. Some means of delivery, such as those used for Rotacaps and Spincaps, may be subject to changes.

Most sufferers or their carers will already know that asthma can be made worse by sudden changes in temperature – either from hot to cold or vice versa. Keep an extra careful watch on young children with asthma if this is likely. Ask your doctor in advance what, if any, increase in dosage of your usual medicines would be wise. Also remember that abroad very different foods may be eaten and, if the sufferer is particularly prone to attack due to dietary changes, try to take a fall-back supply of known, safe foods.

If you feel your asthma or your child's is suddenly getting worse while on holiday, do get in touch with a doctor.

ASTHMA AND PREGNANCY

Having asthma should not put you off having children and in most cases the possible risk of complications, such as high blood pressure, will be no different from any other pregnant woman. However, with severe asthma, as with any other severe condition, it is well worth seeking medical advice before starting a baby.

Women often ask me about the possible risks involved with taking asthma medicines when they are pregnant. Generally speaking, inhaled asthma medicines can be taken while you are pregnant and while you are breastfeeding, but you should always discuss this with your doctor in order to put your mind at rest and to make sure your asthma is managed efficiently while you are pregnant. If you are pregnant and have asthma it is helpful to inform your midwife and hospital staff when necessary, including the anaesthetist in case you need an epidural for pain relief or a Caesarean section. Hopefully the pre-natal exercises should not trigger an asthma attack.

Asthma and pregnancy did worry Elizabeth, a thirty-six-year-old word processor operator, when she was pregnant for the first time four years ago. She had suffered from asthma since the age of five and had come to terms with her condition, but pregnancy posed a new set of worries.

> I have suffered with asthma from as far back as I can remember – I can even remember

my first attack because I was taken into hospital. I recall being put in an oxygen tent, which even though I was only five I didn't find frightening at all. The thing about asthma is when you have a bad attack all you care about is being able to breathe properly again and the oxygen tent helped me do that.

Since that time I have taken a Ventolin inhaler and found that it has helped me control my asthma. I worked out that feathers would aggravate my asthma, so would horse hair, animal fur, household dust or if I had a fright, say if I tripped and fell down. So I always felt confident about avoiding the trigger factors whenever I could and always having my medicine close at hand.

Elizabeth admits this confidence lessened when she realised she was pregnant and her breathing began to be affected almost immediately.

I was worried about taking asthma medicine. My doctor told me I could inhale Ventolin as long as I didn't take it too often and over-dose myself. I felt it was better to take my medicine when I felt the need rather than pass out because I couldn't breathe properly. I also felt confident because I made sure any medical staff such as the community midwife and the midwives in hospital knew that I was asthmatic.

When I first conceived my chest was very wheezy and tight for the first few weeks –

almost all the time. I am just pregnant for the second time, only eight weeks, and the same thing happened again. I had a suspicion a few weeks ago that I was pregnant and then when I started having to get up in the middle of the night to go to the loo and also at the same time my chest began to get bad again, I was certain that I had to be pregnant and I was right.

With the first pregnancy, after the fifth or sixth week my chest got better. I used my inhaler when I had to, when I felt as if I hadn't got any air. I was worried about the last few months of pregnancy when I would be so heavy and the baby would be pushing up on to my diaphragm in case I wouldn't be able to breathe. Some of my friends who had been pregnant always seemed to be breathless at this time and they didn't even have asthma. Yet, to my surprise, at this stage in the pregnancy my asthma was really good. In fact my chest was worse in the very first few weeks of pregnancy than it was in the final few.

Most of my friends told me they were worried about all sorts of things to do with their labour, but I was worried about having an asthma attack when the time came. I had read that it's not common for women to have an asthma attack during labour because their hormones usually prevent it, but I was still worried all the same. But again I was fine. I didn't have time during my labour even to remember that I had worried about how my chest would be!

My chest seemed to be much better for a

long time after the baby was born. I began to notice my asthma started to get worse when he got older at about the age of two and he started to get very heavy. Carrying him on some days made my chest tight but that was something I just got on with.

I've spoken to my doctor about my asthma now I'm pregnant again, although I do feel more relaxed about it second time around, especially as I know that I took Ventolin with no problems at all during my first pregnancy.

Elizabeth's experience of having a worsening asthma experience when she became pregnant is not universal. The increased hormone levels that pregnancy brings have an inflammation dampening effect so that many, if not most, women find that their asthma decreases.

However, later in pregnancy, the baby growing in the abdomen can hamper normal breathing abilities and so produce more distressing asthma symptoms as a result.

ALTERNATIVE TREATMENTS

Most practitioners of unconventional therapies prefer the use of the term 'complementary' medicine rather than 'alternative' because they feel their treatment should work side by side with more conventional methods. No responsible alternative practitioner would suggest that they have the treatment and the cure for all human ills, including asthma. If traditional medicine is not helping, particularly in terms of dealing with stress or emotions, you have nothing to lose by talking to alternative practitioners.

The National Asthma Campaign has pointed out, however, that some trials have shown that acupuncture can relax and might protect against exercise-induced asthma, but it doesn't seem to be particularly helpful in the long-term management of the condition. As for hypnosis and relaxation, techniques such as yoga could be of benefit by helping to relieve stress.

If you do try an alternative therapy, go to a practitioner who is approved by their professional organisation, if there is one. (If there isn't, then consulting them is probably not advisable.) Also, make sure that they are insured against negligence and that you can afford their fees, since you'll have to pay in most cases. Do keep taking your preventative therapy and don't go if your doctor has advised against it.

So what's available? Examples are:

ACUPUNCTURE

Acupuncture has been an accepted form of treatment in China for around 5000 years and these days more and more people in the West are turning to it. Many people believe it is extremely effective in easing a wide variety of conditions by – in simple terms – stimulating the patient's own healing responses.

Traditional acupuncture is a 'holistic' form of medicine – a philosophy which not only treats the symptom but also aims to improve the total well-being of the person. Practitioners believe that many physical conditions can be aggravated by, or are even due to, emotional stress, unsuitable diet, and other factors. So your first visit to an acupuncturist will probably include detailed questions about your lifestyle and a thorough examination. The tongue is especially important in making a diagnosis so don't be surprised if this is carefully examined.

Acupuncture aims to correct any disharmony within the body, to achieve a balance between Yin and Yang. An imbalance, they say, can lead to disease. There are different traditions of acupuncture but they all revolve around the basic principle that the body has an intricate network of linking pathways, 'meridians', which carry our vital 'energies' through the system. These cannot be seen but can be detected using special techniques and can be likened, though loosely, to the nerve pathways known to Western doctors.

During acupuncture very fine needles are inserted into several 'acupoints', according to the problem being treated. By inserting needles or by using pressure, the correct flow and balance of energies can be restored. One theory is that acupuncture stimulates the brain to produce endorphins, the body's natural painkillers.

HOMOEOPATHY

Homoeopathy is a system which works on the theory that 'less is more' and that like cures like. Symptoms are treated by giving a minute dose of a substance which, if given in larger quantities to a healthy person, would actually cause those symptoms.

Even in conventional medicine this principle is sometimes used – for instance, concentrated and controlled doses of radiation are given to destroy cancer cells, which can themselves be caused to develop when too much radiation has been received by normal tissue.

No one has so far been able to explain exactly how homoeopathy works, however, as it does not conform to our accepted knowledge of scientific medicine, though one theory is that during homoeopathic treatment a form of radiation energy is released which stimulates the body's own healing mechanisms. Homoeopaths point out that we don't understand how many modern drugs work either. The disadvantage with these modern drugs though is that we do know that a few have unpleasant side-effects, while homoeopathic medicines don't.

When a person has tried other conventional approaches homoeopathic treatment may be sought. As a holistic therapy (a therapy treating the whole person) part of the treatment process involves a detailed background-taking and people do find that this alone can be a form of counselling.

The aim of this history taking is to match the remedy to the individual patient.

HERBAL MEDICINE

'Herbs' (which include a variety of plants, flowers and even trees) have been used for thousands of years to cure or prevent disease and even today eighty-five per cent of the world's population is largely dependent on herbal medicine. Like homoeopathy, herbal medicine aims not just to treat a particular symptom, but to improve the overall physical and mental well-being of the patient. Diagnosis and treatment based on this holistic approach will include advice on diet and lifestyle, as these may be partly responsible for the symptoms. Herbal medicines may also be used to treat irregular periods, fibroids, ovarian cysts and endometriosis among other problems. In fact, herbalism takes so many factors into account that two people with apparently identical symptoms may be given quite different prescriptions.

Medicines are usually given in the form of a 'tincture' – a concentrated solution made from suitable herbs which have been soaked in water and alcohol. Sometimes the herbalist provides the actual plants from which to make an 'infusion' (similar to tea) or a 'decoction', whereby the plants are gently simmered for some time and the juices then strained off. Medicinal herbs can also be given as suppositories, ointments and poultices.

The herbs used by the herbalist in the treatment of asthma are, in alphabetical order; coltsfoot, elecampane, Euphorbia (also called the asthma weed), grindella lobelia, senega and wild lettuce.

It is likely that all the herbs have a relaxing effect upon the asthmatic tightening of the small muscles which surround the lungs' smaller airways. They may also dampen the inflammation of the airways' lining which also occurs with asthma.

REFLEXOLOGY

The origins of reflexology can be traced back thousands of years and the technique is thought to have been used by the Ancient Egyptians. The art of foot reflexology that we use today was established in the 1930s by an American therapist called Eunice Ingham.

Reflexology works on the understanding that there are areas, called reflex points, on the feet and also on the hands, that match up with each organ, gland and structure of the body – the sole of the foot is thought to represent a map of the body. The spine's reflex point is along the inside edge of both feet which is supposed to be similar in shape to that of the spine. The four arches of the spine – cervical, thoracic, lumbar and sacral – are reflected in the four arches of the feet.

A treatment of reflexology can last around thirty to forty minutes and is likely to involve a variety of massage techniques using the thumb and index finger in addition to a way of rotating the foot, called reflex rotation or pivot-point technique. The technique is a gentle one and many people find it quite pleasurable and relaxing. It is considered that the main benefit is its powers of relaxation, which can relieve stress and tension. It is also said to restore balance, to improve blood supply and to encourage the unblocking of nerve impulses.

YOGA

Yoga has been practised in India for centuries as a means of maintaining mental and physical health. Don't rush into things if you start a yoga class, take things slowly but surely.

Yoga, being a traditional therapy for both toning and relaxing the body's muscles, also relaxes the central and autonomic nervous systems – the latter is responsible for the contraction of the small muscles around the lungs' airways which will contract in an asthma attack. Yoga also has a calming effect upon the emotions – another potential source of relief from emotionally induced asthma.

ALEXANDER TECHNIQUE

Another alternative therapy which could help you deal with stress efficiently is the Alexander Technique. This is a gentle method aimed at relaxing muscles and improving posture by undoing bad sitting and standing habits. An Alexander Technique teacher can point out to you tension you weren't even aware of and how you trigger off this tension at the thought of movement, and instruct you on how to prevent this. Most importantly, the teacher improves your awareness of your body so that you can recognise tension before it builds to the point of causing muscle pain.

OSTEOPATHY

Osteopathy began in the 1870s in the United States and it lays its main emphasis on the structural and mechanical problems of the body. In other words, the osteopath is most concerned with correcting faults in the musculo-skeletal system which is made up of the bones, joints, muscles, ligaments and connective tissue.

Osteopathy is the most orthodox of the unorthodox therapies. It believes that many diseases are due to parts of the skeleton being misplaced and should consequently be treated by gentle methods of adjustment. The General Council and Register of Osteopaths describes the treatment as the 'science of human mechanics'.

Osteopaths use a variety of techniques, ranging from gentle massage or stretching movements to manipulation. It is thought that osteopathy could help chest wall muscle spasm. In people suffering from asthma gentle manipulative techniques are sometimes used to restore proper rib movement and to promote nasal breathing. Gentle relaxation to all the deep spinal muscles is used to promote good relaxation.

Osteopathic treatment tends to be pleasant and relaxing and tailored to suit the needs of the individual concerned. This is why when you first visit an osteopath you will be thoroughly questioned about your medical history.

CHIROPRACTIC

Chiropractic is a method of healing based on manipulation of the spine. Surprisingly, it isn't especially well known despite being the third largest healing profession in the world, after medicine and dentistry. It is a manipulative therapy similar to osteopathy. Chiropractors believe that most problems occur because of misalignment – or 'subluxation' – of one or more of the vertebrae which, they say, can irritate, pinch or cause pressure on a nerve, resulting in pain or other symptoms. And since the spine is the body's primary form of support as well as the channel for the spinal cord and the nervous system, back and spinal difficulties can lead to discomfort and pain in many other parts of the body.

Osteopathic treatment tends to include more soft-tissue techniques (various types of massage) and indirect rather than direct ways of adjusting (manipulating) the affected joints. There are many similarities in the methods used by osteopaths and chiropractors and neither treatment includes any form of surgery and very rarely drugs, which greatly enhances their appeal to many people.

Chiropractors claim that many conditions can respond to this type of treatment including asthma, period pains, back pain, shoulder and arm pain, hip and knee problems, even headaches.

COMMON QUESTIONS

Can asthma be psychological?
People often ask me whether asthma can be due to a nervous disposition. The answer to this question is, no, asthma is definitely not 'all in the mind'. But having said that, your mind can affect the way you cope with asthma and sometimes anxiety can even bring on an attack as sensitive breathing tubes may react to emotional stresses just as they do to irritants you breathe in.

Can asthma be worse at different times of day?
Many people find that their asthma is worse at night than during the day. However, if you find your asthma is disturbing your sleep or you wake early in the morning feeling wheezy or short of breath, it could mean you need more treatment. Do discuss the problem with your doctor. This is especially important in older people, since it can mean that their heart may be under strain.

Can a woman's menstrual cycle affect her asthma?
As with the symptoms that many women experience at the time of the menopause, hormonal changes in the body can result in a wide range of symptoms. If you suspect that your menstrual cycle affects your asthma, keep a diary of the changes you notice. If after several months a consistent pattern emerges, then it is probable that your hormones are behind it.

Can you modify your own medication?
People with asthma do modify their own medication to a certain extent because of the nature of the medicine. Only you know when you need to take your reliever, for example. However, once you've established, together with your doctor, a regular regime of using your inhaler or inhalers – both the relievers and the preventers – it is likely that your symptoms will be kept under control with little modification until, again with your doctor, it may be decided to reduce the frequency of use.

As with any other prescribed medication you should not modify your asthma medication without the advice of your doctor or asthma nurse. Almost all medicines will do you harm if taken in too great a quantity or incorrectly. So follow instructions on the label and your doctor's advice.

Does asthma get worse with age?
Strangely enough, while asthma in children affects twice as many boys as girls, the difference in the sexes is lost as children approach adulthood. Yet in the elderly the difference returns and asthma again becomes more common in men than in women. The trouble with asthma is that it can start at any age. And for those who have had asthma for a long time they may notice a slight difference in symptoms as they get older. Air capacity does depend on age; for instance, a younger man will be able to breathe in more air than an older one. In general, asthma does not deteriorate seriously as we get older.

If you have had asthma once are you always at risk of having it again?
Well, if it really was asthma and not straightforward bronchospasm, then you may have a

tendency to asthma and you can't be sure that you won't have it again. However, bronchospasm is a condition where the small muscles of the breathing tubes quickly contract in response to some severe irritant. As a small boy, several decades ago now, I went into a small and very old-fashioned car battery factory. Inadvertently, I walked into the part where the concentration of sulphuric acid in the air was incredibly high and I couldn't breathe momentarily. I had suffered acute bronchospasm, which fortunately I have never had again. But as a result I can personally appreciate what distress the symptoms of acute asthma must be for a serious sufferer.

Can asthma be cured?
There is no cure for asthma unless a single trigger can be found and avoided. But the symptoms of asthma can be effectively controlled with medication.

I am currently taking steroid tablets for my asthma. My doctor tells me this is short-term treatment. What does she mean?
When asthma symptoms are not readily controlled by inhaled steroids – preventers – and your usual reliever inhaler, doctors may feel the need for a short course of steroid tablets to help control asthma. They are taken over this short period in quite large doses in order that they fully quell the attack, but the dose is then reduced and can often be run down completely so that any potential side-effects can be avoided. Especially in the mainland European countries, quite large doses of steroids are given by mouth for just five days and then stopped abruptly. This seems to control the symptoms quickly and without undue side effects. It is

not so commonly used in Britain, however, in this way. The likely reason is that British doctors are more wary of steroids than our continental colleagues.

My children have asthma but they would love a cat. Should I refuse?
It really does depend upon whether your children's asthma is made worse by the presence of cats. If you have found that in other cat-owning people's houses your children's symptoms start or get worse, then it's likely that another kind of non-triggering pet would be best.

I suffer from asthma and I cough more than other people. Why should this be so?
In a person with asthma, the breathing passages become inflamed, swell and produce excess mucus and also go into spasm. These three factors block the free passage of air in and out of the lungs. It is the restricted movement of air as well as the production of excess mucus which will cause you to cough more than someone who does not have this problem. It is nature's way of trying to rid you of the excess mucus.

How long does an attack of asthma last?
The duration of an attack depends on the individual. Some attacks can last a matter of minutes, while other sufferers may find an attack lasts several hours or days.

Can foods or drinks trigger attacks?
The role of food in an allergic reaction like asthma is cause for much debate. Some people find that certain foods, such as peanuts, and fizzy drinks,

such as lemonade, can make them cough and wheeze. It is far more common for asthma to be brought on by things we breathe in rather than things we eat. However, in my teens I had a friend who suffered quite badly with asthma. His mother tried to see if there was any one food that, when avoided, stopped his asthma. When she excluded eggs or any food that contained them from his diet, his asthma stopped completely. Now that may have been no more than coincidence – his asthma, as it can, was perhaps due to clear spontaneously and naturally. However, I still remember what a relief it was for all of us, not just my friend, when he remained asthma free.

Can food additives trigger asthma?
It does seem that the food additive tartrazine may cause an asthma attack in those susceptible. Tartrazine (E102) is a yellow food dye which, together with a dye called sunset yellow, have been blamed for allergic reactions such as skin rashes and even asthma. It is found in sweets and soft drinks, although more and more manufacturers are labelling their products tartrazine-free as this food dye has also been linked with hyperactivity in children. So if you can avoid it, it is probably best that you do so.

Can exposure to chemicals at work trigger asthma?
There are about 200 or more substances which could cause asthma. One example is a type of material used as solder flux in the electronics industry. Another – which, as I have already explained, caused me to have bronchospasm, one of the asthmatic symptoms – is the vapour given off

by sulphuric acid, and there are many other strong and volatile chemicals which can cause the same reaction.

What's the difference between asthma and chronic bronchitis?

Breathlessness due to asthma usually responds well to treatment, so it is called 'reversible'. However, in conditions such as chronic bronchitis and emphysema, the sufferer – more often a man past middle age – is constantly short of breath to some extent, particularly on exertion. They have what is known as chronic obstructive airways disease (COAD). This is caused by some continual irritation of the airways over many years, nearly always from cigarette smoking. Although the damage, once it has occurred, is not reversible, often much can be done to relieve the symptoms and prevent them getting worse.

In chronic bronchitis, the bronchi and smaller tubes have become permanently inflamed and consequently their damaged and swollen lining isn't able to clear its mucous secretions, which become sticky as they concentrate and may become infected. This sputum has to be coughed up, since the normal clearing processes are hampered by the damaged lining of the breathing tubes. The breathlessness is caused by the struggle for air to get in and out of the lungs through the narrowed bronchi.

What is brittle asthma?

This is quite a rare type of asthma which is very severe. What it means is that the person may appear not to have any symptoms and yet almost in minutes can have a full-blown asthma attack.

Do I need to take asthma medication indefinitely?

Once you have asthma you are likely to have the tendency for life. This means that your asthma can be worse at some times and better at others. Because of the variability in asthma, medication will also be variable. Your doctor will be just as keen as you are to reduce your treatment if the circumstances are right, and just as keen to step up treatment when circumstances dictate the need. But whatever you do, don't stop taking your asthma medicines without the advice of your doctor.

What should I expect from treatment?

With proper treatment most asthmatics will be able to live a normal and fulfilling life, with little time lost from school or work and will also be able to take part in sport.

Can asthma deaths be prevented?

It is a sad fact that even though our understanding and treatment of asthma has improved dramatically, some 2000 people a year still die because of it. In some cases better treatment and perhaps speedier treatment could well save lives. According to the National Asthma Campaign eighty per cent of asthma deaths could be avoided.

Can atmospheric changes trigger asthma?

Atmospheric changes are well-known asthma triggers. Some sufferers have found that thunderstorms can bring on an attack, though it is difficult to be sure why. It would be too easy to say that it is due to the increased humidity. However dry air, especially when it's cold, can also trigger asthma. It may be that some sufferers' asthma is triggered by an increased humidity and for others it's the reverse. It could be due to the sense of foreboding that many people suffer with a storm and any strong emotion may bring on an asthma attack in the susceptible. In short, there's still a lot we don't know about the detail of asthma triggers.

I am a twenty-eight-year-old man and have recently developed asthma. Will it affect my sex life?
My only advice is to continue to take your medication, as advised, and see. The potential excitement and the stress that often accompanies a new sexual relationship may well be the emotional trigger to an attack. However, sexual activity within a secure and loving longstanding relationship may not do so.

Can you tell me what cyanosis is?
Cyanosis is the medical name for the blue tinge which can be seen on the reddest parts of the body in particular – the lips and the nail beds – but all over as well, when the blood is not getting enough oxygen.

I've always had the same medicine for years. Now my doctor has changed it to a generic one which she says is just the same. What does this mean?
A generic is the name used for a medicine that is named by its chemical or scientific name rather than its brand name – the name given to it for marketing purposes by the pharmaceutical manufacturers who have made it.

The increase in generically prescribed medicines

is just part of a change that has been developing as part of the new, cost-conscious NHS, since branded products are usually, though not always, more expensive. If you've been receiving prescriptions for medicines fairly frequently over the last few years, you may have already noticed that the 25,000 GPs in the UK are often prescribing by the generic forms of drugs rather than by brand names. Nearly half of all prescriptions currently written are generic and that proportion is steadily rising. With the NHS reforms and the introduction of fund-holding practices, GPs are having to become price conscious when it comes to prescribing. As I've said, a generic is supposedly the non-branded equivalent of a proprietary, branded drug. Invariably, it is low cost, as generic suppliers only bear the direct cost of manufacture, without the risks of new product development or the costs of gaining the drug's acceptance by doctors. This is a serious cause for concern in the pharmaceutical industry. Also, many manufacturers would claim that the preparation that bears their brand name – and carries the responsibility and benefits of their reputation – is better produced and subject to greater quality control checks than the equivalent generic product.

Should I discuss any side-effects of my asthma medicine with my doctor or should I just ignore them?
Along with its needed effects, a medicine may cause side-effects. You should always discuss side-effects with your doctor and let him or her know if you feel unwell or have any unusual discomfort which you do not understand after taking your medicine.

I have taken salbutamol (Ventolin) for a year now but I don't understand what it does. Can you explain?

Ventolin is a commonly used asthma symptom reliever. The active ingredient is a bronchodilator called salbutamol. This reduces spasm and narrowing of the small air passages in the lungs, making it less difficult to breathe. It also cuts down on feelings of chest tightness and wheezing.

Can you tell me what a rhinovirus is?

A rhinovirus is the name given to those viruses which, in particular, infect the nose in preference to other potential sites of infection – the throat or lungs, for example. They can and do infect other sites however. The many common cold viruses are rhinoviruses.

My doctor tells me I have twitchy airways. Can you tell me what he means?

I think he means that your breathing tubes are particularly reactive to trigger factors for asthma. To be sure, why don't you ask him when you next see him.

ASTHMA RESEARCH

Even as this book goes to print, researchers at London's famous Guy's Hospital are finding that asthma sufferers may have a 'rogue' in-built trigger within the cells of their lungs. Sufferers appear to have an extra protein within these cells which triggers up to fifty times the body's output of other proteins called cytokines, which are responsible for the changes that cause an asthma attack. If this is confirmed, drugs to de-activate this trigger will no doubt be sought.

A spokesperson for the National Asthma Campaign is reported as having said that the findings could ultimately lead to treatments which would stop the process responsible for fatal attacks. A positive point to finish on, I'm sure you'll agree.

USEFUL ADDRESSES

UNITED KINGDOM

The British Allergy Foundation, St Bartholomew's Hospital, West Smithfield, London EC1A 7BE. Tel: 0171 600 6127. Set up in 1991, the British Allergy Foundation is the first national charity concerned with every type of allergy, including hay-fever, asthma, perennial rhinitis, childhood eczema, nettle rash and food allergy. Its aims are to increase the awareness and understanding of allergy as well as provide funds for research projects. Helpline: 0171 600 6166. The helpline is available from Monday to Friday, 10 a.m. to 3 p.m., when you can speak to an allergy nurse. If you would like more information, send a large s.a.e. stamped to the value of 38p to the above address.

The British Lung Foundation, 8 Peterborough Mews, Parsons Green, London SW6 3BL. Tel: 0171 371 7704. The British Lung Foundation was launched in 1985 by a group of chest doctors to raise funds for vital research into lung disease, and to make people aware of the extent of lung disease and the importance of good lung health.

The Department of the Environment's Pollution Helpline, tel: 0800 556677 (calls are free). For information on air pollution levels across the country, health ideas and ideas on how you can reduce pollution.

The Holiday Care Service, 2 Old Bank Chambers, Station Road, Horley, Surrey RH6 9HW. Tel: 01293

774535. Provides information about holidays for those with disabilities, such as asthma.

The National Asthma Campaign, Providence House, Providence Place, London N1 ONT. Tel: 0171 226 2260. Asthma Helpline 01345 01 02 03 (calls charged at local rates).

The helpline is staffed by trained asthma nurses and offers advice and counselling to asthma sufferers and their carers. It is open weekdays from 9 a.m. to 9 p.m. The campaign's aims are to fund research, build awareness about asthma and how it is treated and to offer support to people with the condition. Its quarterly newspaper explains scientific discoveries and new treatments. Its local branches provide personal and practical support.

AUSTRALIA

The National Asthma Campaign, PO Box 360, Woden, ACT 2606, Australia. Tel: 06 282 3265.

CANADA

Association Pulmonaire de Quebec, 3440 Avenue de l'Hotel de Ville, Montreal, Quebec H2X 3B4, Canada. Tel: 514 845 3129.

The Lung Association, National Office, Suite 508, 1900 City Park Drive, Gloucester ONK1 J1A3. Tel: 613 747 6776.

INDEX

acupuncture 82
addresses 100–1
Alexander technique 86
allergic reactions 5
alternative medicine 81–8
antibodies 5
aspirin 58
asthma: age, effect of 90; awareness 63; causes of 4–6; childhood *see childhood asthma*; control of 60–6; cure, lack of 91; diagnosis 7; different times of day, worse at 89; families, running in 19; further medication, requiring 16; genetic factors 6; increase in 17–19; management 8–9, 61–4; meaning 3; number affected by 17; psychological 89; recurrence, risk of 90–1; symptoms 4; treatment 1, 7–12; triggers *see triggers*
asthma attacks: comfortable position, getting into 14; dealing with 12–15; emergency, becoming 15–16; keeping calm 13; length of 92; medical assistance 14; treatment, not responding to 14
atmospheric changes 95–6

beta-agonist 11
beta-blockers 59
breathing difficulties 1
brittle asthma 94
bronchial tubes 3
bronchodilators 8

chemicals, exposure to 93
chest infections: trigger as 6, 58
childhood asthma: advice on 23–5; attacks, dealing with 22; emotions triggering 21; family life, impact on 25; growing out of 1, 20; keeping child informed 27–9; management of 22; numbers suffering from 21; parents, guilt of 24–5; puffers, access to 22–3, 66; school, informing 22, 26, 65–6; severity of 20; symptoms 20–1; triggers 21
chiropractic 87–8
chronic bronchitis 94
cold air, avoiding 75
complementary medicine 81–8
coughing 92
cyanosis 96

deaths, preventing 95
diagnosis 7
doctors: dealing with 60–6; instructions, following 72
drugs: generic 96–7; keeping at hand 69; modification of 90; pregnancy, during 77; protectors 60; side-effects 97; taking as directed 69; taking indefinitely 95

emotions as trigger 21, 45–8
exercise: swimming 40; taking 73; trigger, as 39–45; wheezing during 40
exhaust fumes 32–4, 38–9

food additives 93

hayfever 54–7
herbal medicine 84
holiday, going on 76
homoeopathy 83
house dust mite: allergies, role in 30–1; getting rid of 31–2; heat, thriving in 31; waging campaign against 67–8
houseplants 71

ibuprofen 59
inhalers 7–8, 11: access to 22–3, 66; correct technique 63–4; environment, harm to 36–7; metered dose 36–7
ionisers 75

mast cells 5, 39
medicines as trigger 58–9
menstrual cycle, effect of 89

nebulisers 12

osteopathy 86–7
ozone levels, increase in 32–4

peak flow meter 7, 52, 73–4
pets 92: asthma attack, triggering 21–2
pollen 18, 36; count 56; minimising exposure to 57–8; trigger, as 54–8
pollution: air quality warnings 35, 73; CFCs 36–7; dealing with 35–6; exhaust fumes 32–4, 38–9; ozone levels, increase in 32–4; sulphur-dioxide 32; tobacco smoke 33; trigger, as 32–9, 71–2
pregnancy: asthma medicine, taking 77; smoking during 51; sufferers, of 77–80
preventative therapy 10–11
prevention 67–75

reflexology 85
research 99

rhinovirus 98
rooms, keeping aired 68–9

salbutamol 8, 37, 98
salmeterol 60
school: asthma problems, informing of 22, 26, 65–6
self-help 67–75
sex life, asthma affecting 96
smoking: avoiding 72; deaths from 49; giving up 49; impact of 54; passive 50; pregnancy, during 51; risk of allergy, increasing 48; trigger, as 48–54, 72
sodium cromoglycate 10
sputum 3
steroids: anabolic 10; children taking 26; corticosteroids 10; effects of 2, 10; inhaled 8–10; natural hormones, relatives of 10; short-term treatment 91; tablets 10
stress: positive 46; trigger, as 45–8
swimming 40

terbutaline 8
theophylline 8
tobacco smoke 33
treatment 95
triggers 2, 6: atmospheric changes 95–6; chemicals, exposure to 93; chest infections 6, 58; childhood asthma 21; emotions 21, 45–8; exercise 39–45; factors, working out 69–72; feathers 32; food additives 93; food and drink 92–3; house dust mite 30–2; houseplants 71; in-built 99; medicines 58–9; pollen 54–8; pollution 32–9, 71–2; reaction to 34; smoking 48–54, 72; spicy food 72; stress 45–8
twitchy airways 98

Ventolin 98

yoga 86